The TOTAL BACK BOOK

DR. JENNIFER SUTCLIFFE

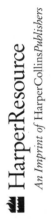

HarperResource
An Imprint of HarperCollinsPublishers

Created and produced by
Carroll & Brown Limited
20 Lonsdale Road
Queen's Park
London NW6 6RD

First published in the USA in 2002
by HarperResource, an imprint of HarperCollins Publishers

Managing Editor Becky Alexander

Editor Kelly Thompson

Designer Roland Codd

Photography Jules Selmes

Library of Congress Cataloging-in-Publication Data has been applied for.

ISBN 0-06-009581-4

The exercises in this book are safe if performed as described, but you should
consult your doctor before beginning this or any other exercise program,
especially if you have an existing medical condition. Neither the exercises nor
the information given with them are intended to replace medical advice. If you
have any concerns about your health, consult your doctor. Neither the author
nor the publishers shall be liable or responsible for any loss, injury, or damage
allegedly arising from any information or suggestion in this book.

Contents

Introduction

Back pain is the most common reason for people taking time off work in industrialized countries, other than colds and the 'flu. Statistics from the University of California show that four out of five Americans suffer at least one episode of back pain during their lives. The reason for this is simple: While the spine is an amazing piece of precision engineering, it has not yet evolved sufficiently to cope with the strains that walking upright places on it.

What can you do when you experience back pain, and how do you prevent it from developing? At one time, bed rest was thought to be the only cure. However, opinions have changed in the last decade, except for in extreme cases. Medical advice now is to continue with your daily activities, including work, but to alter your lifestyle to incorporate good back care. And good back care is what this book is all about.

The Total Back Book explains how the back functions, why you feel different types of pain, and how you can prevent such pain from occurring, or recurring. It contains general advice on how to keep your back in shape, as well as hints on what to do if sudden pain strikes. It also provides you with a series of exercises to integrate into your daily life, according to your particular back type, health problems, fitness level, and lifestyle. Follow these step-by-step exercises, along with the useful hints and tips, and you'll not only start to get your back in shape, but you'll also start to feel fitter, stand prouder, and appear more confident in your everyday life.

HOW TO USE THIS BOOK

Make sure you take time to read the opening pages thoroughly before attempting any exercises. Pages 4–13 are a guide to performing the movements safely and effectively, and will teach you how your back works—making it clear exactly why these exercises are good for you. You'll also learn some technical terms that will be useful for the exercise descriptions later—although they can be found in the glossary at the back of the book, too.

Use the information in Getting Started (page 12) to help you establish which exercises will best suit your needs. However, it is helpful to look through the whole book, in particular the Main Exercises, before beginning, so that you can make a fully informed decision as to which ones to do. Then open the book at the first page you require, unfold the stand onto a nearby surface, and you're ready to start.

What is Back Pain?

The back is one of the most complex and versatile parts of the human skeleton. The key to many of your vital functions (see box, right), it has great strength and flexibility. However, this means that great demands and stresses are placed on it during your daily activities, making it one of the most vulnerable parts of your skeleton. As many of you will already know, it is, therefore, an all-too-common site for aches and pains.

BACK PAIN

Pain is your body's way of telling you that something is wrong. When you have back pain, you experience a sensation generated by the brain in response to signals from pain receptors in your skin, organs, muscles, and other tissues. The intensity of the pain you feel is not due to the strength of such messages, but rather their number and frequency.

ACUTE VERSUS CHRONIC PAIN

Pain messages are of two natures: acute and chronic. "Acute" travels at 10 meters (30 ft) per second, while "chronic" travels at only about 1 meter (3 ft) per second. Acute pain is the more intense of the two as more acute signals than chronic ones can be sent in the same length of time.

Acute pain in the back is usually specific with a recognizable cause (see page 9) and a particular treatment. Chronic pain (see page 10–11), however, can be difficult to explain—even a medical examination can reveal nothing amiss. This is because even very minor damage to the joints, muscles, ligaments, and nerves of the spine can cause pain. The exercises and advice in this book will guide you in how to alter your lifestyle in order to help alleviate chronic problems over time, and prevent any recurrences (see pages 10–11).

IMPORTANCE OF RELAXATION

Endorphins are the "feel good" hormones that your body produces during periods of exercise and positive mental outlook, which override the sensation of pain. When you are tense or anxious, endorphins are not released in adequate quantities to relieve your pain. It is therefore important to remain as relaxed as possible at all times so that enough of them are released. Seek advice from your doctor if any problems arise.

FUNCTIONS OF THE SPINE

- Provides the body with structure to maintain its upright posture
- Supports the head
- Allows movement forward, backward, and sideways
- Protects the spinal cord—the extension of the brain that runs down the spine
- The intervertebral disks act as shock absorbers
- The intervertebral bodies store red bone marrow, which forms blood cells, and minerals
- Provides attachments for muscles and ligaments
- The thoracic vertebrae (see page 6) provide points of attachment for the ribs

The Back's Structure

The spine is made up of 33 vertebrae, although some are fused together so that there are only 26 separate bones. The column is divided into different sections of vertebrae (see below). Understanding how your spine functions will help you keep it in healthy, working order.

JOINTS

Vertebrae are connected to their neighbors by two facet joints, and an intervertebral joint. The surfaces of the small facet joints are covered in cartilage and bathed in synovial fluid, which is all contained within a joint capsule. The fluid in the capsule enables the two bones of the joint to glide over each other without friction. Regular, moderate exercise will keep these lubricated.

An intervertebral joint is composed of two vertebral bodies and an intervertebral disk. The intervertebral disk is a pad that acts as a shock absorber, allowing the spine to move, lengthen, and shorten by molding itself into the required shapes. The inside of it—*nucleus pulposa*—is made of a gooey substance that is 85 percent water; while the hard outside—*annulus fibrosus*—is composed of rings of tough cartilage. These disks can lose a lot of their fluid during a day's activities, so adequate bed rest must be taken to allow their recovery at night.

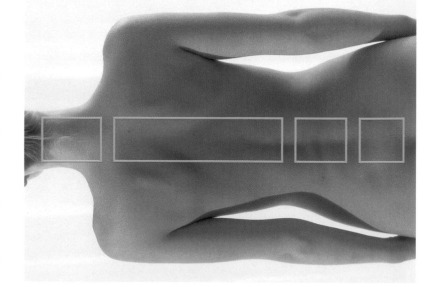

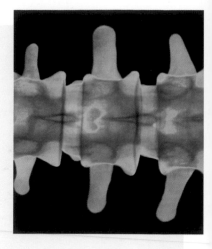

The spinal column is divided into 5 types of vertebrae. These are (from the top down): 7 cervical; 12 thoracic; 5 lumbar; 5 fused sacral; and 4 fused coccygeal (not shown).

WHAT IS A VERTEBRA?

A typical vertebra is composed of:

- A cylindrical mass of bone called a vertebral body that transmits your body weight down the spinal column, and is separated from the next vertebral body by an intervertebral disk.

- A point of attachment for your back muscles and ligaments called the spinous process—the knobs you can see and feel on your back.

- A transverse process on each side, both of which provide points of attachment for your muscles and ligaments.

- Four facet joints—two above and two below that connect each vertebra to the one above and below it.

- A neural or spinal arch running through it—a bony ring that houses the spinal cord.

SPINAL CORD AND NERVE ROOTS

The spinal cord relays sensory information, such as pain messages, from the body to the brain, which then sends orders back down to the muscles to act. It is part of the central nervous system, and runs from the base of the brain, down the neural canal in the spine, to the lumbar vertebrae. Two nerves branch off the spinal cord between each vertebra—one on each side. Back disorders that are particularly painful involve the spine pressing on these nerves, or on the spinal cord itself.

neck and shoulders are known as *trapezius* muscles. The *glutei* muscles in the buttocks support the lower back and pelvis.

Muscles always operate in pairs, so for every muscle that contracts—"agonist," there is an equal and opposite one that relaxes—"antagonist." It is the muscles of the abdomen that work in this way with the muscles of the back to maintain the spine's natural curves. There are four main groups of abdominals ("abs")—the straight abs that bend and flex the spine, two sets of oblique muscles that flex and twist the trunk, and the transverse abs that keep the abdomen's contents pulled in. You should exercise all back and stomach muscles equally so that there is no danger of muscular weakness or imbalance, which can lead to back pain.

MUSCLES

The spine is supported and moved by an intricate network of muscles. There are three main layers of muscles in the back. The small inner layer connects each vertebra to its neighbor; the middle layer connects groups of vertebrae; and the large outer layer—the *erector spinae* muscles—connect the whole spine from top to bottom. The large muscles that work the

LIGAMENTS

Ligaments are broad bands of tough tissue that bind the vertebrae together, allowing the spine to move as one piece. There are two long ligaments, which run down the length of the spine at the front and back of the vertebral bodies, as well as small ligaments binding each vertebra to its neighbors. Ligaments have a poor blood supply, and do not heal easily if strained or torn.

The spinal cord (blue and yellow) is an extension of the brain. It relays sensory information to the brain from the rest of the body, relays orders from the brain to the muscles, and is protected by the vertebrae of the spinal column (white).

It is important to keep your stomach muscles strong, as well as your back muscles, because your spine can't function without them to relieve strain. The straight abs (left) and the external obliques (right) are shown as blue outlines.

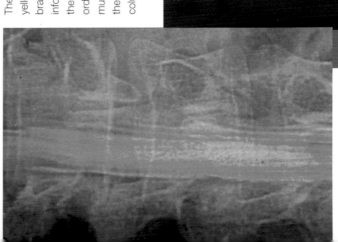

Importance of Good Posture

When viewed from behind, the spine is a straight line in the middle of the back. When viewed from the side, however, it should appear curved. The thoracic and sacral vertebrae curve backward. They are known as primary curves as they are present at birth. The cervical and lumbar vertebrae, on the other hand, curve forward, and develop as a baby learns to raise his head, and sit up. It is these natural curves that give your back the ability to maintain your upright stance, as well as the resilience to absorb the downward forces of gravity, your body weight, and the impact from the ground as you walk or run. The single most important way to look after your back is to maintain this natural posture (see right).

POSTURAL PROBLEMS

If your back is held too straight, or over-arched, the spinal column cannot cope with everyday stresses, and may start to malfunction. This may affect the order in which you should do the steps of certain exercises. Using the points below as a guide, check and see whether you have any postural problems:

- Flat back—an overly-straight, rigid back.
- Hollow back or lordosis—an exaggerated concave arch in the lower back.
- Rounded shoulders or kyphosis—an exaggerated convex arch in the back, giving a hunchback appearance.

Always strive to maintain good posture, not only when standing, but also when sitting, moving around, and during exercise. See pages 18 and 20 for additional information.

TIPS FOR CORRECT POSTURE

- Aim to have the crown of your head, rather than the top of your forehead, as the highest point of your body.
- Your head, neck, and chin should be kept in a neutral position—neither jutting out nor tucked too far in.
- Relax your shoulders.
- Neither arch nor slouch your back, thus allowing it to maintain its natural curves.
- Pull in your abdominal muscles.
- Try to keep your pelvis slightly "tucked" under.
- Keep your knees slightly bent, and your feet hip-width apart, and pointing forward.
- If stationary for a long period of time, keep shifting your weight from one foot to the other.
- If standing at a work surface, adjust its height if possible so that you do not have to bend over too much.

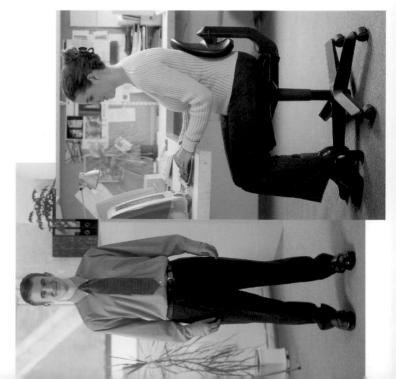

Acute Back Pain

The intense, unpleasant, and often very sudden sensation of acute back pain can be localized to one area of the back, or can radiate down the arm (brachalgia) or leg (sciatica) if a nerve root is compressed. Most episodes of acute back pain are the result of a flare-up of a chronic back problem. Just one incorrect or sudden movement, for instance, may cause a prolapsed disk, facet joint inflammation, or a torn ligament if the back or stomach muscles are weak. Chronic degenerative conditions, such as osteoarthritis and osteoporosis, can also reach such a degree that they cause acute pain.

PROLAPSED—OR "SLIPPED"—DISK

Standing, sitting, and bending put immense pressure on the intervertebral disks. If you don't have adequate support from your muscles and ligaments, a disk may bulge out to the side, or into the spinal canal. The disk does not "slip" as such as it is firmly attached to the vertebral bodies, but rather the *nucleus pulposa* leaks out through a crack in the *annulus fibrosa*, causing local muscle spasm and pain. If the bulge happens to press on a nerve root, severe pain can be felt not only in the back but the whole length of the nerve (see Sciatica, pages 80–81).

FACET JOINT INFLAMMATION

These small joints that hook the vertebrae together can become inflamed if the bones are squashed too tightly together, or if they are pushed out of alignment by a sudden pressure. The joint capsule then swells causing local pain,

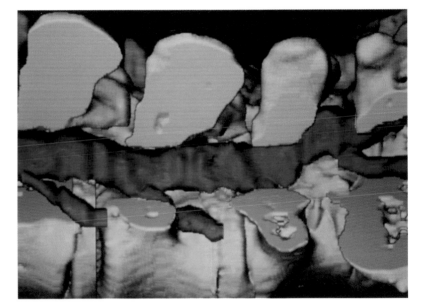

which may radiate to other areas if the swollen capsule presses on a nerve.

CENTRAL CANAL STENOSIS

In this disorder, the spinal canal that contains the spinal cord narrows. As the spinal cord is very sensitive to pressure, even a slight narrowing can cause severe pain and other neurological symptoms (see box, below). The main causes of central canal stenosis are being born with an abnormally small spinal canal, suffering a prolapsed disk, or having osteoarthritis (see pages 82–83), where bony spurs (osteophytes) protrude into the canal.

This scan shows a prolapsed disk (green, lower center) pressing against the spinal cord (blue). The disk's outer layer has weakened, allowing its contents to spill out, causing pain and possibly numbness.

EMERGENCY ACTION

If you hurt your spine in an accident or fall, you may experience neurological symptoms such as numbness, or "pins and needles," which may be the result of a fracture, or dislocation of a vertebra. Make sure you keep absolutely still, as any movement could cause paralysis. Call for emergency medical assistance.

Chronic Back Pain

One of the most common complaints in the Western world, chronic back pain is largely due to postural faults and a sedentary lifestyle. What causes the pain is often not fully understood, as even minor injuries to the soft tissues, muscles, ligaments, and joints of the spine can result in an intermittent or constant ache. However, some of the main causes are discussed below.

POOR POSTURE

Any habitual posture that changes the spine's natural curves (see page 8) can cause chronic pain. It is important to try to correct poor posture before it starts to "feel" natural, as the muscles and ligaments can adapt, but the spine cannot. The unequal pressures on the spine—one muscle group becoming overstretched while its opposing muscle group becomes lax—can cause the disks to harden and lose their elasticity, the facet joints to become compressed, and can even hasten the onset of osteoarthritis. To improve your posture, follow the advice on page 8, and throughout the book. If postural problems persist, consider utilizing the Alexander Technique (see page 89).

MUSCULAR WEAKNESS

The spine needs support from both abdominal and back muscles so that an even and equal pressure can be maintained throughout the length of the vertebral column. Weak abdominal or weak back muscles do not contain enough tension to do this. If the back muscles are stronger than the abdominals, as is common, ligament strain and joint damage can occur at the front side of the spine. Regular performance of the exercises in this book will help keep your muscles strong on both sides of the body.

MUSCULAR IMBALANCE

Most people do not use both arms to the same degree. As a result, the muscles on one side of the body become more developed than those on the other. Even a minor difference in strength can affect the joints of the thoracic spine: the small muscles on the stronger side can become too tense, the ligaments lose their flexibility, the disks become compressed, and the facet joints jam together. In extreme cases, this can lead to scoliosis (pages 84–85). You can help prevent muscular imbalance by adopting correct posture, starting all exercises on your weakest side, and either wearing a backpack with the weight distributed equally over both shoulders, or alternating the side on which you carry your bag or briefcase.

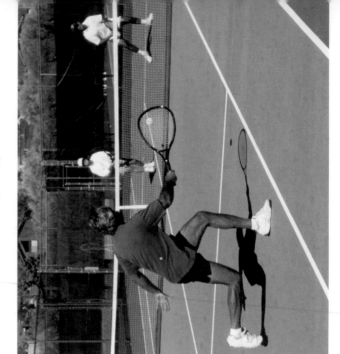

One-handed sports like tennis can lead to muscular imbalance. The exercises in this book will help strengthen the muscles on the underused side of your body.

SEDENTARY LIFESTYLE

Muscles, ligaments, and joints need to be used regularly to stay healthy. Movement not only maintains muscular strength, but carries vital nutrients to your body's tissues. Without movement your intervertebral disks dry up and shrink, your facet joints become impacted, and your ligaments lose their elasticity. Lack of exercise is also likely to lead to an increase in bodyweight, putting extra strain on the spine.

Taking regular, gentle to moderate exercise plays a vital part in keeping the muscles, ligaments, and joints of your back in healthy, working order.

LIGAMENTS AND FACET JOINTS

A strained or torn ligament can be a source of both acute and chronic pain as it takes a long time to heal properly. An overstretched ligament may weaken and no longer adequately control your movements, while an underused ligament may become stiff. Take particular care with your movements if you have recently had a ligament problem as damaged ligaments are especially vulnerable to further injury. Facet

joints are also extremely susceptible to damage and may flare up with misuse.

DEGENERATIVE CONDITIONS

Progressive disorders, such as osteoarthritis (see pages 82–83), or osteoporosis (see pages 86–87), may be a likely cause of any chronic pain, the older you become.

Ankylosing spondylitis—or "bamboo spine" — is another degenerative disorder, which mainly affects young men. A hereditary disease, the first sign is stiffness and chronic lower back pain in the morning. As the disease progresses from the base of the spine to the neck, the vertebrae gradually fuse together, and the intervertebral disks and ligaments harden until the spine forms a rigid forward bow.

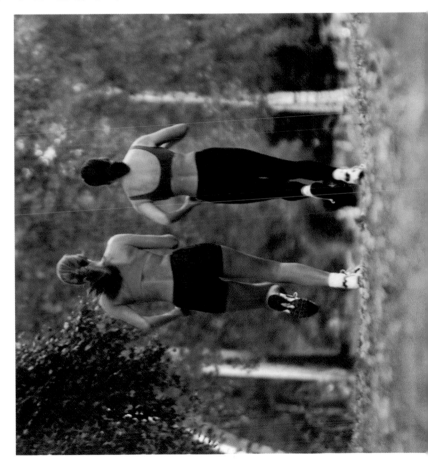

Getting Started

The purpose of this section is to make sure you and your back get the most from the exercises in this book. It is vital to choose the exercises that suit you best, and to listen to your body throughout all movements. Have everything you need at hand (see box, right). You can vary the number of exercises you do in your program according to your fitness level, and the time available to you. Work at your own pace.

Read all the exercises before beginning as this will familiarize you with the full range of possibilities, and allow you to make an informed decision as to which ones are best for you. However, if time is short, here are some short-cuts you can take to help you:

- Read the "Is it right for me?" panel on the top page of each exercise.

- Establish whether you have any basic postural problems (see page 8), as this may affect which exercises you do, and the order in which you do them.

- Use the Rescue Plan (pages 14–17) to work out which exercises may be the most suitable starting points for you.

- If you suspect or know you have a condition that appears in the Problem Backs section (pages 80-87), look there first, as advice is given on which exercises to attempt first.

- Read the "Purpose" panels and choose at least two abdominal exercises, one exercise that extends your back, and one exercise that rotates the spine as part of your program.

- Watch out for any "Caution" boxes. These warn if an exercise is unsuitable for you.

You probably will find that quite a few exercises are suitable, so try varying the elements of your program from time to time to build up your repertoire, and to prevent boredom.

WHAT YOU WILL NEED

- Adequate space and privacy
- Loose comfortable clothes, and sneakers that fully support your ankles
- An exercise mat, available in most sports stores—to protect your spine when doing exercises lying down
- A comfortable, upright chair that lets your feet touch the ground
- Water—to prevent dehydration
- Two small towels for use in certain exercises
- Strap-on wrist weights—as an optional extra to increase the difficulty level when you are familiar with the exercises

BE AWARE

Consult your doctor before doing back exercises if you suffer from:

- cardiovascular disease
- a neurological problem
- osteoporosis
- severe arthritis, especially in the neck
- episodes of dizziness

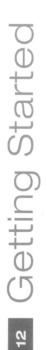

MAKE BACK CARE A HABIT

Regular performance of the back exercises in this book will keep you supple and pain-free, improve your posture, and increase your general sense of well-being and self-esteem.

Set aside time—about three times a week—when you can spare an hour to give your back a good work-out. On other days, just do a few of the simple stress relievers, such as the office stretches (see pages 18–21).

You should wear loose-fitting clothes and shoes that support your ankles when doing any sort of weight-bearing exercise.

FIND YOUR OWN LEVEL

If the Main Exercise seems difficult, complicated, or even just awkward for one reason or another, start with the "Easy Alternative." With practice, your strength and flexibility is likely to increase enough to progress to the Main Exercise. Then, once you are confident with it, use the "Progression" to add to your sequence, or to replace it altogether.

THE NEXT STEP

It is essential that you complement your exercise program with general back care. Develop realistic strategies to incorporate good posture and activity into your daily life, like walking to work, or taking one yoga class per week. See page 92 for further suggestions.

LISTEN TO YOUR BODY

If you are experiencing back pain that does not subside with movement or changes of position, the cause of the pain may not be spinal. Non-spinal causes include problems as diverse as: inflammation of the pancreas or gallbladder; gallstones; kidney infections or kidney stones; cardiovascular problems; influenza; meningitis; and benign or malignant tumors. Cease doing the exercises, and contact your doctor immediately.

EFFECTIVE EXERCISE TECHNIQUES

- Always do the Warm-Up Exercises (see pages 22-33) before the Main Exercises.

- Read all instructions carefully.

- Make sure you do an "Essential Follow-up" when there is one.

- Know your own limits, and choose the level of exercise that best suits you. Never force a movement or position.

- Do all exercises in a slow and controlled manner, especially when rolling and unrolling the vertebrae.

- Maintain good posture throughout the exercises (see page 8).

- Remember to breathe deeply throughout all exercises.

- At the end of your exercise program, you should allow your spine to return to a neutral position by relaxing on the mat for a few minutes.

- Stop exercising immediately if you experience any pain, feel faint, or become dizzy, or short of breath. Slow down if you are breathing heavily, and feel overheated.

Rescue Plan: Acute Pain

Whether you experience extreme pain all of a sudden or it is built up over time, you need to deal with it right away. Answer the questions below to find a suitable course of action. However, the information in this chart should not replace the advice of your doctor.

Are you experiencing extreme, sharp pain that has come on suddenly?

OR

Have you experienced pain recently but it has now become more extreme and sharper?

YES

YES

Have you lost weight, had a temperature, or been feeling tired?

NO

Is your pain worse after standing or walking, but less on bending or leaning forward?

NO

YES

YES

Possible non-spinal causes (see page 13 for list)

SEE YOUR DOCTOR

Possible central canal stenosis (see page 9)

SEE YOUR DOCTOR

EMERGENCY RELIEF POSITIONS

If you find the exercises recommended in the flowchart uncomfortable, adopt one of the three emergency relief positions below:

Lie flat on your back, breathe deeply, and relax as much as possible.

Lie on your back and raise your bent legs to rest on a comfortable surface.

Lie on your stomach, with your head to the side that provides the most relief.

If your pain does not subside or improve within 48 hours, see your doctor as soon as possible.

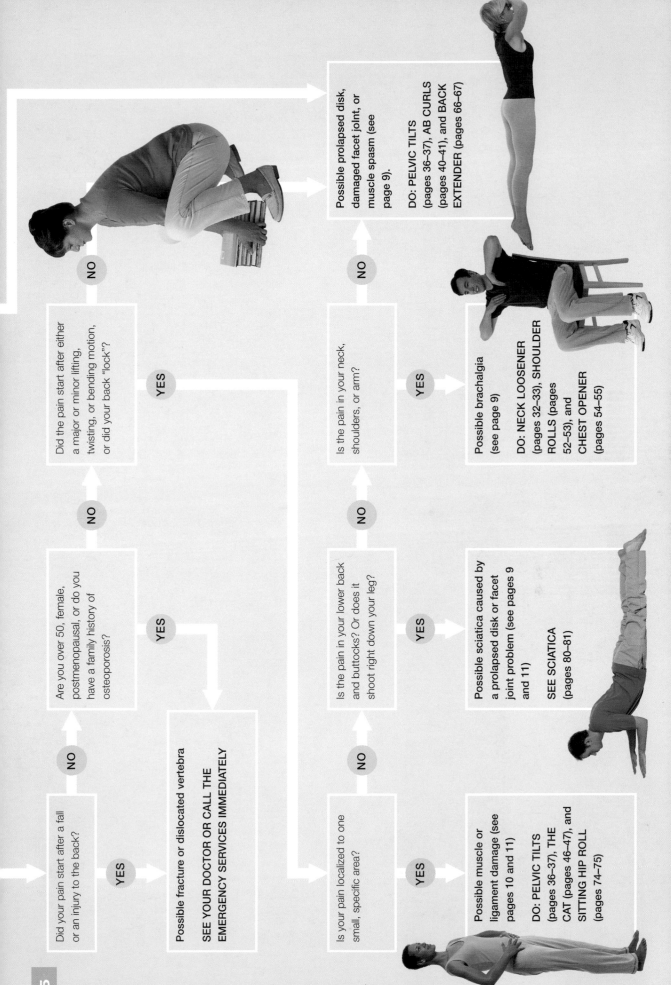

Did your pain start after a fall or an injury to the back?

NO → Are you over 50, female, postmenopausal, or do you have a family history of osteoporosis?

NO → Did the pain start after either a major or minor lifting, twisting, or bending motion, or did your back "lock"?

NO → Possible prolapsed disk, damaged facet joint, or muscle spasm (see page 9).

DO: PELVIC TILTS (pages 36–37), AB CURLS (pages 40–41), and BACK EXTENDER (pages 66–67)

YES (from fall/injury) → Possible fracture or dislocated vertebra

SEE YOUR DOCTOR OR CALL THE EMERGENCY SERVICES IMMEDIATELY

Is your pain localized to one small, specific area?

NO → Is the pain in your lower back and buttocks? Or does it shoot right down your leg?

NO → Is the pain in your neck, shoulders, or arm?

YES (neck) → Possible brachalgia (see page 9)

DO: NECK LOOSENER (pages 32–33), SHOULDER ROLLS (pages 52–53), and CHEST OPENER (pages 54–55)

YES (lower back/leg) → Possible sciatica caused by a prolapsed disk or facet joint problem (see pages 9 and 11)

SEE SCIATICA (pages 80–81)

YES (localized) → Possible muscle or ligament damage (see pages 10 and 11)

DO: PELVIC TILTS (pages 36–37), THE CAT (pages 46–47), and SITTING HIP ROLL (pages 74–75)

Rescue Plan: Chronic Pain

When you suffer from ongoing back pain, it is difficult to know how to lessen discomfort, and prevent further trouble. Answer the questions below to find a suitable plan of action. However, the information in this chart should not replace the advice of your doctor.

Have you experienced aches and pain in your back for a considerable time?

YES

Is your pain accompanied by other symptoms, like tiredness, weight loss, or a high temperature?

YES

Possible non-spinal causes (see page 13 for list)

SEE YOUR DOCTOR

NO

Does your pain become worse in cold weather, after activity, and/or in the morning?

YES

Possible muscle spasm or ligament strain caused by general factors like poor posture, and muscular weakness or imbalance

ANY OF THE EXERCISES IN THIS BOOK WILL HELP YOU REGAIN STRENGTH IN YOUR BACK

NO

Does your pain become worse after sitting, standing, or leaning forward for long periods of time?

NO

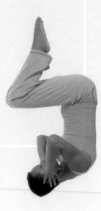

Possible abdominal weakness (see page 10)

DO: AB CURLS (pages 40–41), HIGH-LEG ABS (pages 42–43), and CROSS ABS (pages 68–69)

RESCUE PLAN: CHRONIC PAIN

Do you have pain in your groin, hip, or down your thigh into your knee?

Do you have pain in your lower back, buttocks, or neck?

Is your pain worse early in the morning but improves with activity?

YES

NO

NO

YES

NO

YES

NO

YES

NO

YES

Possible ankylosing spondylitis (page 11)

DO: BACK OPENER (pages 44–45), THE CAT (pages 46–47), and BACK EXTENDER (pages 66–67)

Possible muscle spasm or ligament strain caused by general factors like poor posture, and muscular weakness or imbalance

ANY OF THE EXERCISES IN THIS BOOK WILL HELP YOU REGAIN STRENGTH IN YOUR BACK

Possible sacral ligament strain (see page 11)

CONCENTRATE ON THE LOWER BACK EXERCISES (pages 66–77)

Are you over 50?

Possible osteoarthritic spine

SEE OSTEOARTHRITIS (pages 82–83)

Are you over 50?

Possible osteoarthritic hip

DO: CROSS ABS (pages 68–69), PELVIC LIFTS (pages 70–71), and SIDE LEG RAISES (pages 72–73)

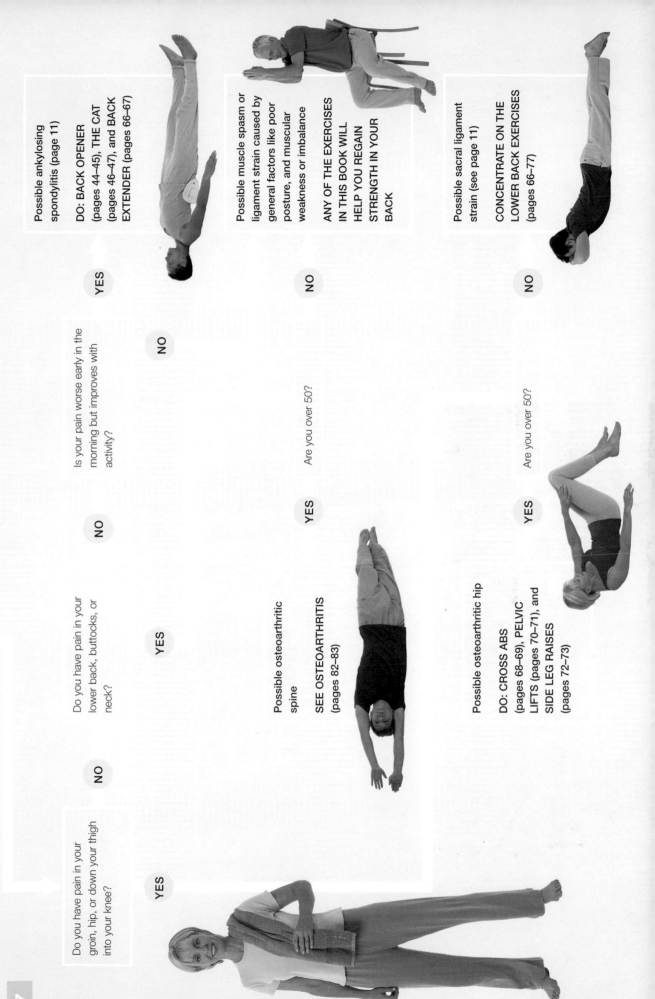

Work Stretches: Sitting

More than ever before, today's workers are desk-bound. This is unfortunate as sitting imposes more strain on the spine than standing or walking, and puts the back under great stress. There are some simple exercises which will help to relieve the pressure.

When sitting, gravity increases the pressure of the upper body's weight on the lower spine. If pressure within the lower spine is considered as 100 percent when standing, it is 150 percent when sitting up straight, and 250 percent when sitting slouched over—emphasizing how crucial it is not to slouch. The intervertebral disks only get a chance to recover when you are lying down, reducing the pressure to 25 percent.

It is therefore very important to make sure your work environment suits your needs. Your chair should be fully adjustable in seat height, angle, and the position of the backrest. You should always try to adopt the correct sitting posture (see right), as well as performing the mini-program of exercises below to relieve any tension. Special back chairs are also available, which redistribute the pressure down the spine, thighs, and onto the knees, thus reducing the pressure in the spine. However, these chairs are not suitable for those with knee problems.

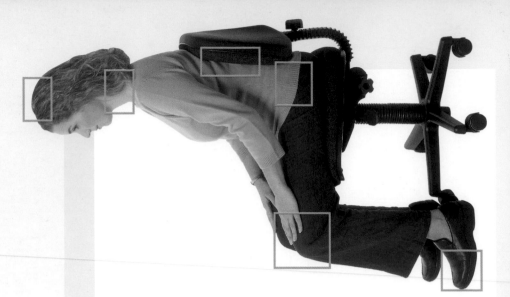

TIPS FOR CORRECT SITTING POSTURE

■ Keep your neck in a neutral position, with the crown of your head as the tallest part of your body.

■ Your backrest should be upright but slightly molded so that it supports the lumbar curve of your spine.

■ Your seat should be wide enough to support your thighs, and either horizontal, or tilted down and forward by up to 5 degrees.

■ Maintain a slight pelvic tuck throughout your working day.

■ Your seat should be at a height that allows your feet to rest flat on the ground, with your lower and upper legs at right angles to one another.

Points to remember at your desk:

■ You should be able to view your computer screen without tilting your head either too far up or down.

■ Your work surface should be just lower than your bent elbows so that there is support when necessary.

■ Your legs should be under the work surface so that you do not need to lean forward to reach the keyboard.

SITTING MINI-PROGRAM

Even if you feel comfortable in your chair, you should always take frequent breaks. Stand, walk around and stretch out your spine five or six times a day. It is also advisable to do a mini-program such as the one below. This will help ease the tensions of your working day.

The exercises shown below are those that are most suitable for performing while in the workplace. They can be found in larger format in the Main Exercises Section. You can add others—depending on which exercises you feel are most beneficial to you. Run through the mini-program at home first, so that you know how to do the exercises correctly. It should take no longer than five minutes. Then try to do the sequence at work, at least once each morning and once each afternoon. If time is short, Pelvic Tilts can be done discreetly and easily throughout the day.

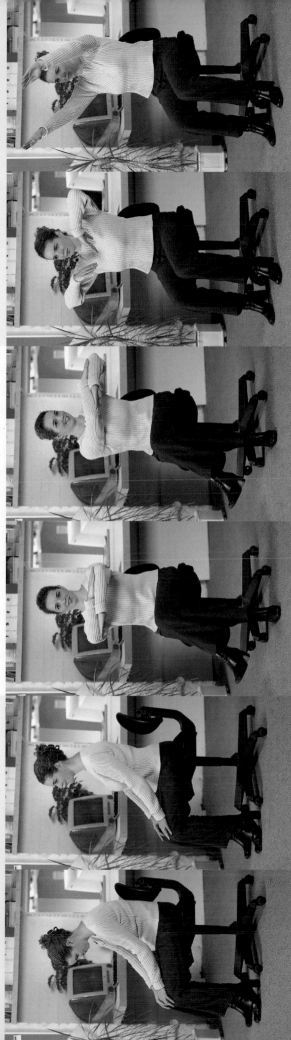

SHOULDER ROLLS (pages 52–53)

Circle your shoulders backward 5 times, then forward 5 times. Repeat with your elbows. Finish by circling your arms backward 5 times.

SPINAL TWIST (pages 48–49)

Cross one leg over the other, and fold your arms at shoulder height. Twist your upper body and head to the left and right alternately 5 times. Repeat wth your other leg on top.

PELVIC TILTS (pages 36–37)

Sink back to sit on the upper part of your tailbone and top of your buttocks. Then sit up tall, arching your lower back so that you are on the tip of your tailbone. Repeat 10 times.

Work Stretches: Standing

Although standing does not put as much pressure on the spine as sitting, it can still take its toll over time. If your job requires you to stand for much of the day, here are some exercises that will help protect your back.

When you stand still for long periods of time, your spinal joints and ligaments receive no increase in blood supply, and no extra lubrication, in contrast to when you are active. The stretched ligaments can become lax, too, offering less support to the spinal joints. If you stand over a work surface, you are likely to be leaning forward as well, further increasing the pressure on your back by making your muscles work even harder. Avoid the aches and pains this can cause by maintaining good posture (see page 8), and by breaking up your day with the mini-program of exercises below.

It is also important that you maintain good posture when lifting and carrying objects—activities that are often required at work. Although any imbalanced and incorrect movements can damage the spine, you are particularly vulnerable to injury when bending, twisting, and lifting, so follow the advice on the right concerning how to lift correctly.

TIPS FOR CORRECT LIFTING TECHNIQUE

- Stand as close as possible to the object to be picked up.
- Adopt a wide stance, with one foot slightly further forward than the other for balance.
- Bend your hip and knee joints to squat down, rather than bending your back.
- Allow your heels to lift slightly off the floor as you become low enough to lift the object.
- Pick up the object as centrally as possible so that the weight is distributed evenly.
- Keep your back as straight as possible as you slowly stand up, using the power in your leg muscles to raise you.
- Keep the object close to your body as you come up to standing position.
- Carry out all movements slowly and with control.
- Never twist and lift at the same time.

STANDING MINI-PROGRAM

Even if you know and understand the theory behind good posture, it is still difficult to "feel" whether you are standing in the correct way when carrying out your everyday activities. It is a good idea to check your posture in the mirror at home so that you can be sure that what you

feel is right is, in fact, correct. Then try to maintain this feeling in your daily life. Even if you are in the habit of standing correctly, it is advisable to do a mini-program such as the one below to ease any tension, and to give your spine a good stretch. You can use it in addition to the Sitting Mini-Program if you wish.

Run through the mini-program at home first so that you are familiar with the exercises. It should only take five minutes. Then try to do it at least once each morning, and once each afternoon at work. The information below is a guide as to what to do, but you should turn to the relevant pages for full exercise descriptions.

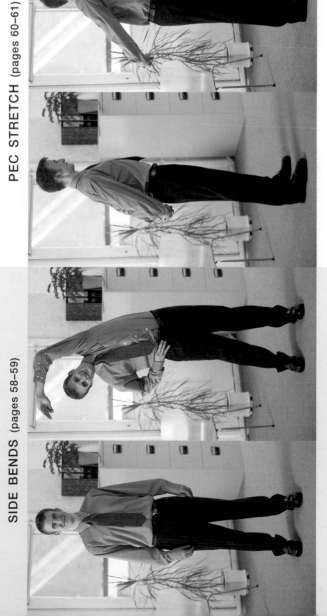

SIDE BENDS (pages 58–59)

Stand with your feet hip-width apart. Put one hand on your waist, stretch the other above your head, and lean over to the side. Keep your lower body still. Repeat 5 times on each side.

PEC STRETCH (pages 60–61)

Clasp your hands behind your back, turn your elbows in toward your spine, and push your arms upward, without leaning forward. Hold for 10. Repeat 5 times.

THORACIC STRETCH (pages 62–63)

With your feet hip-width apart, hollow your back as much as possible, and hold for 10. Repeat 5 times. Then round your back as much as you can, and hold for 10. Repeat 5 times.

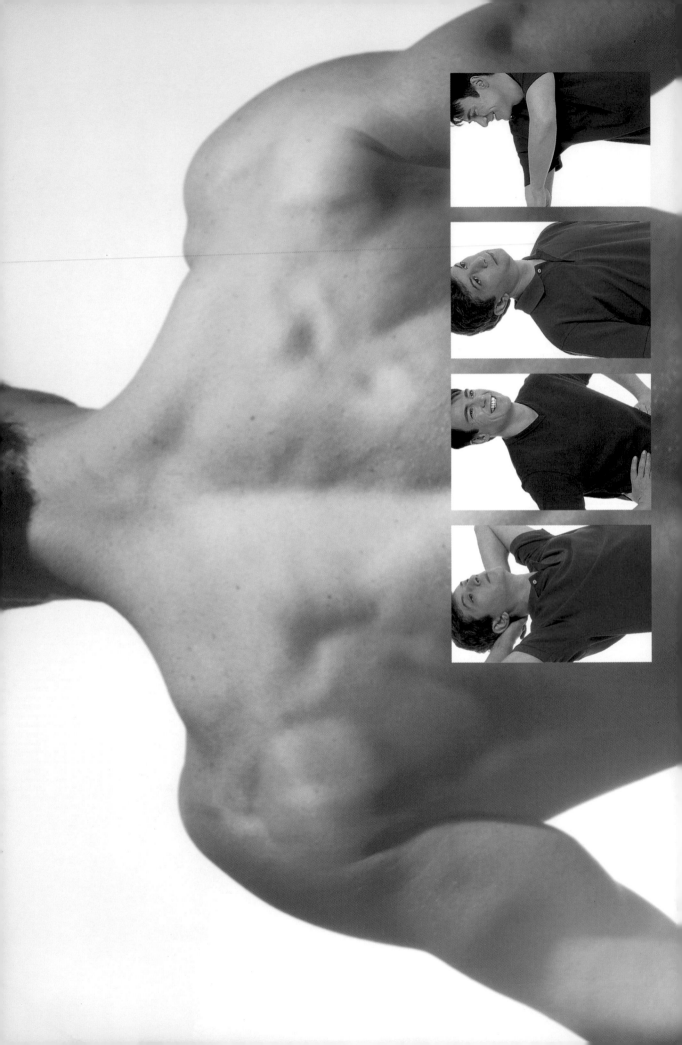

Warm-Up Exercises

It is essential you do the exercises in this section before performing any of the Main Exercises (see pages 34–77). Warm-ups not only prepare your muscles, joints, and ligaments for the more demanding activity to come, thus reducing the risk of injury, but they also increase the effectiveness of the Main Exercises.

The short sequence of Warm-Up Exercises will not take long to perform; allow yourself fifteen minutes. It is important both to start and finish the sequence with Spot March and Jog in order to adequately increase your heart rate, as well as to loosen all relevant body parts.

The general aims of the exercises are to:

- loosen the joints, and flex the ligaments in preparation for the Main Exercises;
- gradually increase your heart rate in order to pump blood—and therefore nutrients—around your body faster;
- raise your body temperature gradually so that there is no sudden increase in temperature when you start the Main Exercises;
- increase the rate of chemical reactions in your muscles, making them more efficient;
- raise the speed at which nerve impulses travel to the muscles so that the body is better prepared for further activity.

Spot March and Jog

During periods of inactivity, your circulation slows down and the blood supply to internal organs is increased at the expense of the supply to the muscles—especially those of the leg, abdomen, and back. Spot March and Jog increases the blood supply to the muscles.

This exercise should always be the first, and last, part of your warm-up routine and you should wear impact-reducing shoes while doing it. Spot March and Jog increases the rate of your circulation and quickens your pulse so that more blood reaches your working muscles. The increased blood supply gives the muscles the extra oxygen and nutrients they need to function efficiently, and also means that the chemical waste products produced while the muscles are working are carried away more quickly.

The extra blood supply has another benefit, too. Tissue fluid passes out of your blood and into your cells, providing important lubrication for the joints, muscles, and ligaments, and rehydrating the intervertebral disks in your spine. This extra lubrication is necessary if you are to decrease the risk of sustaining any muscle and ligament injuries, or joint sprains.

Start all exercises slowly, only gradually building up intensity. However, this is even more essential in the warm-up stage as the whole aim of this section is to get your body accustomed to this new activity.

If you prefer, you can replace jogging on the spot with other exercises that will increase your heart rate, such as ski jumps, where, each time you jump, you land with one leg and the opposite arm forward.

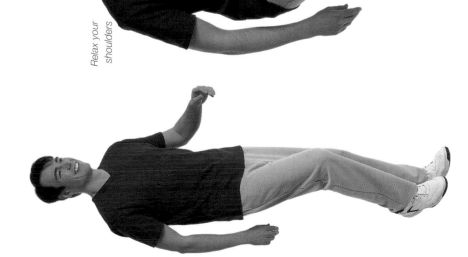

Relax your shoulders

Keep your back straight

Place your heels down each time your feet land.

1

Stand tall, and tighten your stomach muscles. Walk on the spot, and swing your arms as if marching, each arm moving with the opposite leg. **Do this for approximately 1 minute.**

2

Gradually start raising your knees toward hip level, adjusting your arm swings so that each hand touches its opposite knee. **Continue for approximately 3 minutes.**

3

Jog gently on the spot for 3 minutes. Raise both hands above your head, touch them to your shoulders, extend them out to the sides, and return them to your shoulders as you jog. Repeat this arm movement. **Finish by repeating Step 1.**

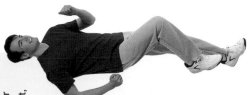

EASY ALTERNATIVE

If Step 3 is too vigorous for you, simply jog on the spot, omitting the large arm movements. Make sure you place your heels on the floor each time your feet land on the ground.

Trunk Stretch and Twist

The muscles that rotate the back, and the joints that they work on are often underused and out of balance as we tend to twist more to one side than the other, depending on which hand we favor. These factors make the muscles vulnerable to sudden stresses. The Trunk Stretch and Twist will help lessen this vulnerability.

PURPOSE

To loosen the spinal joints and ligaments, the muscles of the ribs and vertebrae, the large oblique muscles of the stomach, and the back muscles, and to increase the blood flow to them in preparation for exercise.

Is it right for me?

This exercise is suitable for people of all back types. It is important that you work at your own level—do not exceed what you are comfortable with.

This exercise rotates and stretches the upper back and lower back in turn, loosening the joints of the shoulders, vertebral column, rib cage, and pelvis in preparation for the Main Exercises later in the book. The Trunk Stretch and Twist trims the waist, too, if carried out regularly.

It is important that you do this warm-up exercise in order to minimize the risk of muscle and ligament tears, and joint sprains when you move on to the Main Exercises. Mobilizing the joints also means that your body will be more comfortable with and accustomed to this style of movement, and will therefore be able to move that little bit further when it comes to working on any imbalances, or weaknesses throughout the Main Exercises.

Do not push yourself too hard while doing the exercises. It is important to notice that you move only the upper body in Step 1, and only the lower body in Step 2. Carry out the movements slowly, making sure you keep within your own limits.

If you prefer, Step 2 of the Trunk Stretch and Twist can be carried out sitting down.

1 Stand tall with your knees slightly bent, and your feet shoulder-width apart. Raise your arms out at shoulder height.

Your feet are parallel

2 Swing your arms horizontally from side to side so that you twist to each side alternately. Keep your arms straight, and your hips as still as possible throughout. **Repeat 10 times in each direction.** Finish with both arms out to their respective sides at shoulder height.

Keep your lower body still

3 Place your hands on your waist, and twist one knee inward by lifting your heel off the ground, and swiveling your toe in toward your other knee. Return to the original position, and immediately do the same movement with your other leg, so that the exercise flows rhythmically. **Repeat the sequence 5 times.**

Keep your upper body still and facing forward

EASY ALTERNATIVE

Sit on a chair with your legs hip-width apart. Bend forward, stretching one hand down toward your opposite foot. Rest your free hand on the chair. Hold for a count of 3, then rise slowly to the starting position. Now stretch your other hand toward your other foot. Repeat the sequence 10 times.

Forward Bend

The ligaments supporting the back often become too tight as we rarely stretch down and forward in everyday life. As a result, they can tear if any sudden movement is made, for example when you bend your back incorrectly to pick something up from the floor. The Forward Bend will decrease the chances of this happening.

This exercise reduces tension in the ligaments and muscles, and stretches out and mobilizes the spine both when it is bent and arched. If you omit it from your warm-up routine there is a risk that a sudden overstretching of the ligaments during the main exercises may cause the muscles to go into a protective spasm, not only causing you pain but also further straining the ligaments.

The Forward Bend is a simple exercise and yet it is often performed incorrectly. Follow each step carefully, and recognize the limits of your own flexibility by bending only as far as is comfortable.

You should not push too far to the floor, or bounce up and down in the bent position of Step 2. The weight of your upper body will stretch the muscles of your back sufficiently as long as you relax properly. Nor should you arch back too far in Step 3. A small movement of 15 degrees is your aim, and this will avoid putting too much strain on the small of the back. It is crucial that all the movements are as slow and controlled as possible.

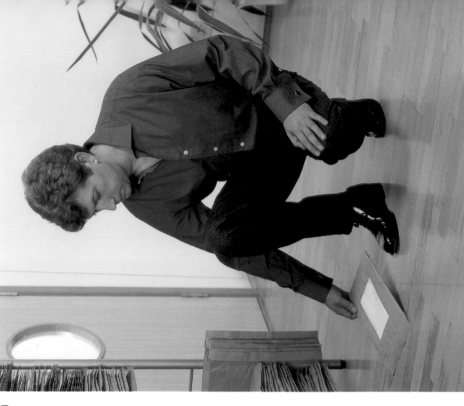

When picking items up from the floor or a low surface, bend down as shown above—bending your knees rather than your back—in order to avoid possible injury.

PURPOSE

To mobilize the spine, to stretch the large muscles of the back, thighs, and stomach, and to open up the rib cage.

Is it right for me?

This exercise is suitable for people of all back types. If you have a flat back, do the exercise as given. If you have a hollow back you should switch Steps 2 and 3 so that you finish the exercise by bending forward.

CAUTION

Do not arch your back more than 15 degrees, especially if you have weak stomach muscles, or neck problems. Be careful not to let your head fall back. Make sure that your knees are not locked as this may strain your lower back.

1 Stand tall with your feet shoulder-width apart, and your knees slightly bent. Tighten your stomach muscles, and make sure your bottom is tucked in.

Relax your shoulders

2 Bend down slowly from your hips until you feel a stretch in your hamstrings. Let your hands fall closer to the floor to stretch your back muscles a little more. **Hold for a count of 30.** Then gradually come back up, vertebra by vertebra.

Your knees are slightly bent

Keep your abs tight

Your chin is in a neutral position

3 Place your hands behind your head to support your neck, and lean back about 15°. Push your elbows back to expand your rib cage, and arch your whole spine—not just your lower back. **Hold for a count of 30,** then contract your stomach muscles to help pull yourself up straight. **Repeat the exercise 3 to 5 times.**

EASY ALTERNATIVE

You may need to do this version if you have neck problems, weak stomach muscles, or a poor sense of balance. Lie down on your side on the floor, and curl up into the fetal position. Hold for a count of 10, then uncurl, stretching and arching your back. Repeat 5 times.

Hip Circle

If you stand or sit still for much of the day, as many people have to do at work, it is likely that the weight of your upper body will compress the vertebral joints of your lower back. This can reduce flexibility, especially when you try to turn to one side or the other. The Hip Circle will help you maintain your twisting flexibility.

PURPOSE

To mobilize the lower back, hips, and thighs, strengthen the abdominal muscles, and relax and stretch the small intervertebral muscles and ligaments of the lumbar spine.

Is it right for me?

This exercise is suitable for people of all back types. It is especially important for those who spend long periods sitting or standing still.

This exercise mobilizes your lower back in preparation for the Main Exercises that help with flexibility, such as The Pilates Roll (see pages 50–51), and Cross Abs (see pages 68–69). It loosens and warms up the small muscles and ligaments that support the spine in the lower back, and also helps firm the abdominal muscles.

Twisting requires small movements at each vertebral joint. All of these small movements combine to produce one whole movement. As it is impossible to target individual vertebrae, the broad, swinging, rhythmic movements involved in the Hip Circle are used to make sure that all the tissues are warmed up.

The thoracic spine has the most capacity for rotation, but this exercise will help you keep all areas of the spine capable of such movement.

A variation of the Hip Circle can be performed on a swivel chair to achieve a similar twisting movement. Allow your knees to drop slightly to one side while your arms reach to the other side.

1 Stand tall with your feet shoulder-width apart, your knees slightly bent, and your hands on your waist. Then tighten your stomach muscles.

Keep your pelvis tucked and your abs tight

Your knees are slightly bent

2 Slowly circle your hips, making sure that your body is kept still above the waist so that the movement is in the lumbar spine, pelvis, and hips only. **Do the movement 10 times**, then repeat **10 times in the opposite direction.**

Keep your head in a "neutral" position

3 Stand as before, but this time keep your body still below the waist. Circle your whole upper body 10 times one **way, then 10 times in the opposite direction.**

EASY ALTERNATIVE

If you find the circling motion difficult to master, practice a "twisting" motion instead. Stand with your feet hip-width apart, and swivel your feet from side to side, wiggling your hips. Hold a towel at either end behind you, and allow it to rub on the top of your buttocks to make yourself more aware of the movement.

Neck Loosener

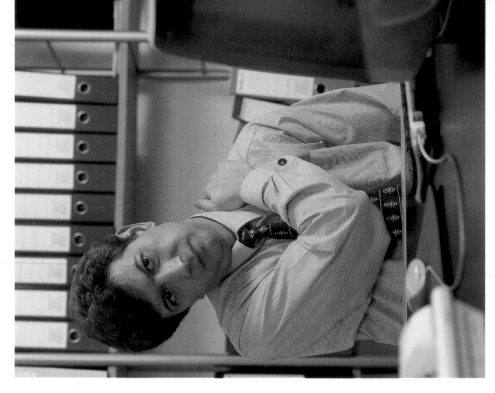

Many people who have rounded shoulders, or who spend most days hunched over a desk, suffer from muscular tension headaches. These are often a sign of shoulder and neck problems, as a combination of bad posture and stress has made your muscles taut and knotted. The Neck Loosener will help prevent such headaches.

PURPOSE

To increase flexibility by loosening the neck and shoulder joints, and to reduce tension in the muscles of this area.

Is it right for me?

This exercise is suitable for people of all back types. It is especially useful for those with hunched shoulders, or who sit at a desk for long periods at a time.

CAUTION

You should not do this exercise if you have a neck problem or suffer from arteritis (inflammation of the arteries) unless you check with your doctor or physical therapist first.

This exercise loosens and eases the muscles and joints of the neck and upper back, and reduces any unnecessary tension in the large muscles of the neck and shoulders. The most important of these muscles are the two large *trapezius* muscles—one running down each side of the neck to the back of the shoulders—where a lot of the tension gathers.

When you are slouched, with your head pushed forward and your shoulders rounded, it means that the neck and shoulder muscles contract in an attempt to prevent you from falling further forward. This nearly static state of contraction causes some of the muscle fibers to go into spasm and form knots.

It is important that you do the Neck Loosener to start easing the knots before doing any of the Main Exercises involving the neck and shoulders. Otherwise there would be a slight risk of the muscles tearing at the site of the knots. An added advantage of the Neck Loosener is that you can do it either sitting or standing, and it is quite relaxing, as well as beneficial.

In addition to being an essential part of the warm-up routine, the Neck Loosener is an ideal tension reliever that you can carry out discreetly any time you feel neck tension building up.

NECK LOOSENER

Relax your shoulders

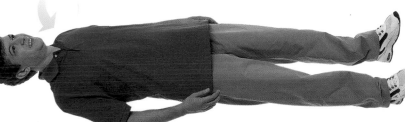

1 Stand tall, and circle both shoulders backward. **Do this 3 times, then repeat 3 times forward.**

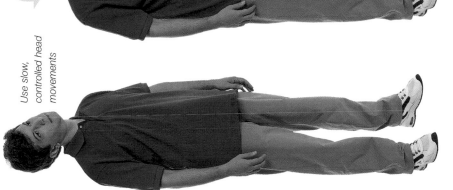

2 Next, keeping your head and shoulders level, turn your head to look first over one shoulder, then the other. **Repeat 3 times.**

Use slow, controlled head movements

3 With your head level and shoulders still, move one ear down toward the shoulder on the same side. Hold for 3, and raise again. **Do this 3 times, then repeat moving your head to the other shoulder.**

Only move your head as far as is comfortable

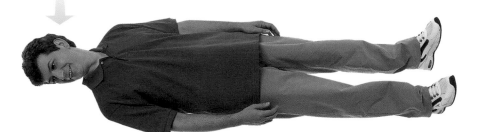

4 Slowly circle your head 3 **times**—to one side, down to your chest, to the other side, and back up to neutral each time. **Repeat 3 times in the opposite direction. Finish the sequence by repeating Step 1.**

ESSENTIAL FOLLOW-UP

Now that your muscles and ligaments have been stretched and your joints mobilized, it is important that you increase your heart rate once more as the final part of your warm-up routine before starting any of the Main Exercises: Return to pages 24–25 to do the Spot March and Jog again.

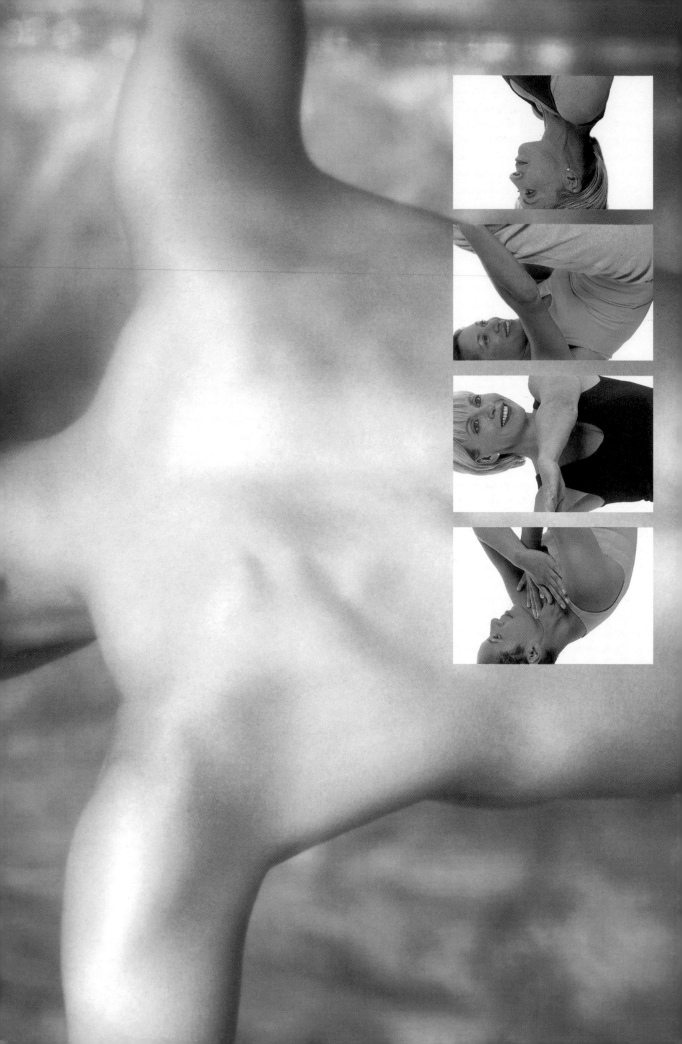

Main Exercises

The exercises in this section are effective both for preventing back problems from developing, and for relieving any existing back pain. They address postural problems, promote muscular strength, improve flexibility, and increase support for your spine.

The majority of the Main Exercises in this section are suitable for everyone, but if you have any specific concerns, read the information provided in the introductory pages, along with the "Purpose," "Is It Right for Me?" and "Caution" boxes on the exercise pages themselves to check if an exercise is suitable for you.

When creating a routine, make sure it is balanced:

- include several Whole Back exercises (pages 36–51) in order to increase your overall strength and flexibility;
- do several Upper Back exercises (pages 52–65), especially if you have hunched shoulders, or

spend your working life sitting at a desk;

- perform several Lower Back exercises (pages 66–77), especially if you spend a lot of time driving, or bending and lifting heavy objects;
- make sure you include some exercises for your abdominal muscles, which provide vital support to your spine.

The directional arrows on certain exercise steps are there to help you see at a glance what the main movements are. Handy tips on posture and effective exercise technique are also interspersed throughout the exercises.

Pelvic Tilts

The bottom of the lower spine takes the weight of the upper body, especially when you are sitting. If this area is either too flat or too hollow, the vertebrae are placed under great stress. The result can be lower back pain and sometimes osteoarthritis in later years. Pelvic Tilts will help prevent this.

PURPOSE

To mobilize the lower back, lubricate the intervertebral disks, reduce lower back stiffness, and correct posture.

Is it right for me?

This exercise is suitable for people of all back types. In fact, it is the most useful of all back exercises and can benefit everyone, whether carried out as an exercise or within everyday movements.

This exercise mobilizes the lower back, and helps to correct an overly straight back or a hollow one.

Although it is not complicated, many people find the movement difficult, especially when the back is unyielding and hollow. It is best to learn the exercise when lying down, practice it when sitting, and then move on to performing it when standing. This will maximize the postural benefit you gain from it.

PROGRESSION

Stand with your feet hip-width apart, your knees slightly bent, your pelvis in a neutral position, and your hands on your hips. Tighten your stomach muscles, and tilt your hips forward, then push them back so that your bottom sticks out. Once the movement starts to feel natural, rock backward and forward 10 times.

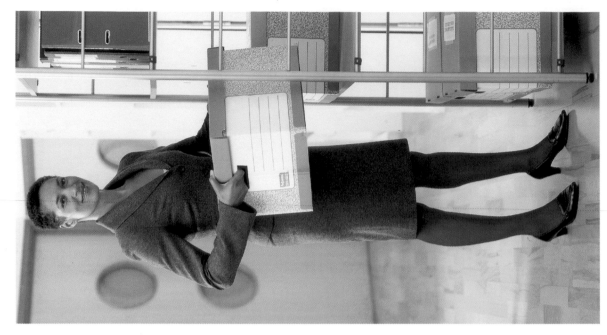

The Pelvic Tilt movement also can be used while performing your everyday activities. Tuck your pelvis in when lifting and carrying objects to prevent damaging your back.

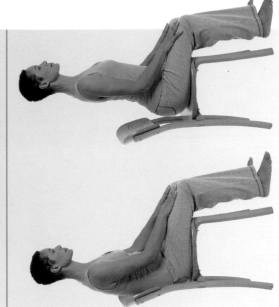

EASY ALTERNATIVE

Sit up straight with your feet on the ground. **Keeping your upper back straight, sink back so that you are sitting on the upper part of your tailbone and the top of your buttocks. Then sit up as tall as possible, arching your lower back forward so that you are sitting on the lower tip of your tailbone and your upper thighs. With** practice you can turn it into a rocking motion that can be used to exercise your muscles when sitting at a desk.

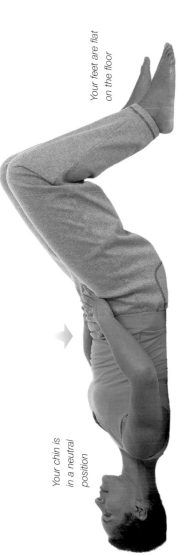

Your chin is in a neutral position

Your feet are flat on the floor

1 Lie on your back with your knees bent and hip-width apart, and your feet flat on the floor. Pull in your stomach muscles, and push your lower back down into the mat. Allow the tip of your tailbone to lift off the mat but keep your upper back still. **Hold for a count of 5.**

Your knees are hip-width apart

Breathe deeply throughout the exercise

2 Arch your lower back up off the floor, and allow your tailbone to tilt down to the mat. **Hold for a count of 5. Repeat Step 1 and 2 movements 10 times** without holding in between so that the movements become continuous. Finish with your spine in a neutral position—neither arched nor flat.

Cross-leg Roll

Many back exercises ignore the rotational and oblique muscles of the back, and the ligaments that support the spine. As a result, these can become tight, reducing your flexibility and making you more vulnerable to injury through sudden movements. The Cross-leg Roll will help prevent any such problems.

PURPOSE

To strengthen and release tension in the rotational and oblique muscles, and improve flexibility by loosening the intervertebral ligaments and joints of the lower back.

Is it right for me?

This exercise is suitable for people of all back types. It is especially useful for those with sciatica (see also pages 80–81). If the sciatica pain runs down the right leg concentrate on crossing the left leg over the right leg, and vice versa.

This exercise focuses on strengthening the neglected rotational and oblique muscles, which make actions like getting out of the car and lifting luggage off carousels in the airport much easier.

People who often sit with one leg crossed over the other are likely to find the Cross-leg Roll easier, because doing so stretches out the ligaments and small muscles in the spine.

PROGRESSION

Take up the starting position as before but stretch your arms out wide at shoulder height, with your palms up. Push your bottom leg down to the side with your top leg, and lift the hand on the same side as the legs over to touch the inside of your other elbow. Hold for a count of 5. Then do this with the other arm and leg. Repeat the whole exercise 4 times.

The Cross-leg Roll Progression twists and stretches the body, making you more mobile and flexible.

1 Lie down with your knees bent and hip-width apart, and your feet flat on the floor. Place your hands behind your head, and rest your elbows on the floor. Pull in your abs, and cross one leg over the other.

Relax your shoulders

2 Keeping your upper body flat on the floor, use the top leg to push the bottom knee down to the side until you feel a stretch across your other hip and lower back. Only stretch as far as is comfortable for you—not to the point of pain. **Hold the stretch for a count of 10, and repeat 5 times.**

Keep your upper body flat on the floor

3 Repeat the exercise sequence with the opposite leg on top, crossing the legs in the opposite direction.

Keep your head in a neutral position

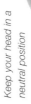

EASY ALTERNATIVE

This is a simpler exercise with a lesser stretch, but one that will still release spinal tension. Lie in the starting position as before, but do not cross your legs. Instead, move both bent legs together over to one side so that the leading leg rests on the floor. Then lift them back up and over to the other side, the leading leg once again resting on the floor. Move continuously from side to side 10 times. Keep your stomach muscles tight throughout.

Ab Curls

The abdominal muscles support the spine, and are essential for good posture. However, most people's abdominals are not strong enough to support the spine properly. Ab Curls will strengthen the muscles so that they can do their job more effectively.

PURPOSE

To strengthen the abdominal muscles so that they can give support to the spine, and maintain correct body alignment.

Is it right for me?

This exercise is suitable for people of all back types. In fact, everyone would benefit from doing some Ab Curls at least three times every week.

This exercise is a variation on the full sit-up, but with bent knees, and only a small head raise. A full sit-up should not be used, because the abdominals are only capable of lifting the chest off the floor to an angle of 30 degrees before the hip flexors contract, putting great strain on the lower spine.

Ab Curls help reduce the stresses placed on your spine during your everyday activities. An additional benefit is that they also trim your waist.

PROGRESSION

Lie as in Step 1, place your hands behind your ears, and raise your thighs to right angles with the floor. Raise your head and shoulders up as before, keeping your lower back flat on the floor, and your thighs still. Hold for 3, uncurl, and repeat 5 times.

You will need to practice the Main Exercise before you are comfortable with this Ab Curls Progression. The more confident you become, the more repetitions you can do.

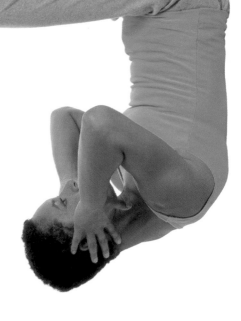

CAUTION

You must perform this exercise in a smooth, controlled manner to avoid straining your lower back, or damaging your abdominal muscles. Only do as many as are comfortable for you.

Your knees are hip-width apart and your feet are parallel

1 Lie on your back with your knees bent and hip-width apart, and your feet flat on the floor. Cross your hands over your chest, and pull in your stomach muscles.

Keep your neck relaxed

2 Raise your head, and curl your upper body up off the mat to an angle of about 30 degrees. Keep your head in a neutral position as you move, and keep the part of your back below your shoulder blades in contact with the floor. **Hold for a count of 3.**

Pull your abs in tight

3 Uncurl your upper body, and lower down, vertebra by vertebra. Start off with approximately 5 repetitions to ensure that the exercise is smooth and controlled. Gradually work up to 20 controlled curls a day.

ESSENTIAL FOLLOW-UP

Use this exercise after your Ab Curls to stretch out the muscles you have been working, and to relieve any stiffness. Lie on your back on the floor with your hands above your head and your toes pointed. Stretch from the tip of your fingers to your toes, elongating your body as much as possible. Hold for a count of 10, relax, then repeat 3 times.

High-leg Abs

If you spend long periods of time on your feet, especially hunched over some kind of worktop, you're likely to experience rounded shoulders, increased tension in your spine, and possibly swollen feet. High-leg Abs will help ease these problems.

PURPOSE

To straighten the back, ease spinal tension, strengthen the abdominal muscles, and aid lymphatic drainage from the legs, thus reducing swelling in the ankles.

Is it right for me?

This exercise is suitable for people of all back types. It is especially useful if you tend to stoop, have weak abdominal muscles, or if your feet sometimes become swollen.

This exercise stretches the whole back, and eases spinal tension. It also strengthens the abdominal muscles, improving posture, and increasing support for the spine.

There is an additional benefit, too. When you walk, or climb stairs, the contractions of your leg muscles push blood and tissue fluid up the leg through the veins and lymph vessels. This process is called the "muscle pump." Conversely, if you stand still for a long time, the muscle pump becomes inactive, allowing tissue fluid to collect in the ankles and feet, and possibly making them swollen. High-leg Abs activate the muscle pump, and also enable gravity to drain tissue fluid away from the feet.

PROGRESSION

Keep your buttocks against the wall at the end of Step 3, bring your hands down to your sides, and stretch one hand toward the opposite ankle, lifting your shoulders off the mat. Hold for a count of 5, then uncurl slowly. Relax, then do this on the opposite side. Repeat this sequence 5 times, and finish with the Essential Follow-Up.

It is best to use a wall as support for the legs during the High-leg Abs Progression, because your muscles may not be strong enough to hold them in this position on their own.

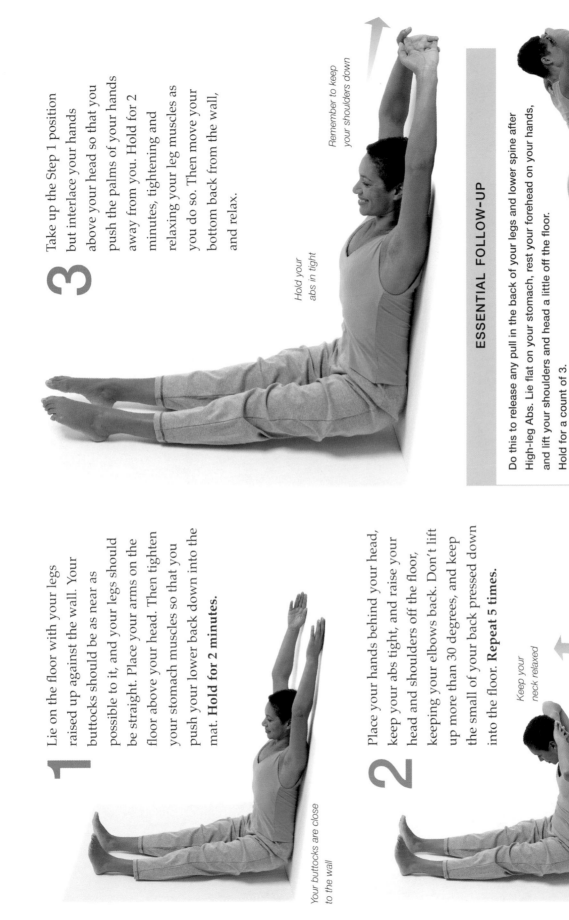

3 Take up the Step 1 position but interlace your hands above your head so that you push the palms of your hands away from you. Hold for 2 minutes, tightening and relaxing your leg muscles as you do so. Then move your bottom back from the wall, and relax.

Hold your abs in tight

Remember to keep your shoulders down

ESSENTIAL FOLLOW-UP

Do this to release any pull in the back of your legs and lower spine after High-leg Abs. Lie flat on your stomach, rest your forehead on your hands, and lift your shoulders and head a little off the floor.
Hold for a count of 3.
Repeat 5 times.

1 Lie on the floor with your legs raised up against the wall. Your buttocks should be as near as possible to it, and your legs should be straight. Place your arms on the floor above your head. Then tighten your stomach muscles so that you push your lower back down into the mat. **Hold for 2 minutes.**

Your buttocks are close to the wall

2 Place your hands behind your head, keep your abs tight, and raise your head and shoulders off the floor, keeping your elbows back. Don't lift up more than 30 degrees, and keep the small of your back pressed down into the floor. **Repeat 5 times.**

Keep your neck relaxed

Back Opener

If you have to stand or sit for long periods of time, your intervertebral disks may start to become compressed, making them lose fluid and shrink. The Back Opener is an exercise that will help counteract any such problem, and will assist in preventing the discomfort it would cause.

PURPOSE

To stretch any tight intervertebral muscles and ligaments, and to counteract the effects of sitting and standing for long periods by opening up the side of the spine nearest the stomach in order to let the disks reabsorb water.

Is it right for me?

This is suitable for people of all back types. It is especially useful for those who lead a sedentary lifestyle or who have a tendency to slouch.

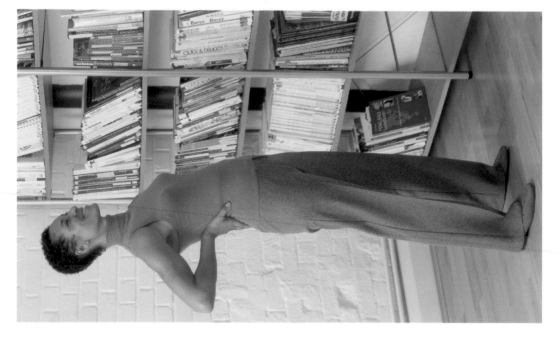

This exercise stretches the intervertebral muscles and ligaments, increasing flexibility. The Back Opener also opens up the side of the spine nearest the stomach, enabling the intervertebral disks to suck in water and expand, making them more capable of their job as shock absorbers. You need a rolled-up towel to do this exercise.

Spinal compression can result in a height shrinkage of as much as an inch during a day of standing. Luckily, the disks reabsorb water during the night when we are lying flat, so that our normal height is restored by the morning. However, while the spine is compressed, the intervertebral joints push down on each other, making the muscles and ligaments tighten, and the spine lose its flexibility.

PROGRESSION

When your back loosens up, you could use a specialist back block instead of a homemade roll to increase the arch of your spine. These are available in many fitness stores.

Put your hands on the small of your back, and gently arch your back to relieve tension after activities that involve bending or stretching, like reaching for an object on a low shelf.

1 Lie on your back with your knees bent and hip-width apart, and your feet flat on the floor. Lift your buttocks up off the floor, and slide a rolled-up towel under your tailbone and hips. Then relax down onto it, keeping your arms by your sides on the mat.

Keep your head in a neutral position

Relax into this position

2 Straighten your legs out so that your body forms an arch over the roll. Then relax completely, and rest in this position for anything from 1 to 10 minutes, depending on how long you remain comfortable.

Keep your knees hip-width apart and your feet parallel

3 Bend your knees again, lift yourself off the rolled towel, and remove it. Then lower your buttocks to the floor, and relax.

ESSENTIAL FOLLOW-UP

Do this after the Back Extender to equalize the stretch on the front and back of your spine. Pull your knees up to your chest, and gently rock them backward and forward 3 times to stretch the spine in the opposite direction from the Main Exercise.

The Cat

During a typical day, moisture is sucked out of the intervertebral disks, reducing the space between them. This increases the chances of wear and tear on the disks, and inflammation of the facet joints. The Cat will help decrease the chances of either problem occurring.

PURPOSE

To spread out the vertebrae so that the intervertebral disks can replace the fluid lost during the day, and to strengthen the muscles that support the spine.

Is it right for me?

This exercise is suitable for people with a normal or hollow back. If you have a flat back, do Step 3 before Step 2.

This exercise strengthens the abdominal muscles, increases the support they give to the spine, stretches out the spine, and opens up the vertebrae so that moisture can be reabsorbed by the disks. An additional benefit is that it is a relaxing exercise to do, as it reduces tension in the *erector spinae* muscles, which run down either side of the spinal column. The Cat is particularly effective if you have been sitting or standing still for a long time.

PROGRESSION

In the arched position of Step 3, take a breath in, then exhale as you sink down to sit on your heels, keeping your head toward the floor. Feel the stretch over your spine, hold for a count of 3, then rise to the starting position.

You can do The Cat Progression on its own as a quick tension-reliever after you have been standing or sitting in the same position for a long time, or as part of your regular exercise program.

EASY ALTERNATIVE

If you have a rounded back and shoulders, try doing this exercise with your fingers pointing toward your knees. This flattens the top of the back. You will only be able to arch up with the lower half of your back.

1 Kneel on all fours with your legs and arms shoulder-width apart, your hips directly above your knees, and your shoulders directly above your hands. Pull your stomach muscles in, and check that your spine is straight. Breathe naturally.

Start the exercise with a flat back

2 Breathe out while you raise your head and hollow the small of your back. Relax your back as far as it will go without causing any discomfort. **Hold for a count of 3.**

Keep your arms slightly bent

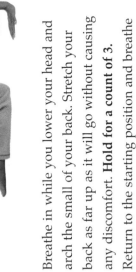

3 Breathe in while you lower your head and arch the small of your back. Stretch your back as far up as it will go without causing any discomfort. **Hold for a count of 3.** Return to the starting position and breathe naturally. **Repeat the exercise 5 times.**

Tuck in your pelvis

Spinal Twist

Many people find it difficult to turn to look behind them because the spine has a limited capacity for rotation. This type of movement becomes even harder if your spine is not regularly utilized. The Spinal Twist helps remedy this problem.

PURPOSE

To increase the spine's range of rotational movement, and to make it equally easy for you to turn in either direction.

Is it right for me?

This exercise is suitable for people of all back types.

This exercise stretches the muscles and ligaments of the whole back, including those of the rib cage, and enhances flexibility so that you can turn easily to either side, or look behind you. It also can counteract the problem that most people have of being more flexible on one side than the other.

The Spinal Twist is beneficial to the thoracic spine in particular, because the thoracic vertebrae have minimal forward and backward movement compared to those of the rest of the spine, but have the greatest capacity for rotation.

PROGRESSION

Do the exercise as before, but uncross your legs and fold them in before trying the extra twist in Step 3 (see right). Push both knees down to the floor, and make sure that the hand behind you remains still.

The movement in the Spinal Twist Progression will help you twist and turn in everyday activities, such as looking over your shoulder while driving.

1 Sit on the floor with your legs stretched straight out in front of you, and your hands down by your side. Bend one leg, and cross the foot of that leg over your straight leg.

Make sure you keep your back straight

Relax your shoulders

2 Bend the opposite elbow to the outside of the bent knee, and rest it along your thigh to prevent your leg from moving.

Your fingers are facing backward

3 Rest your free hand on the floor behind you. Then turn your head and body to look behind you. Hold for a count of 10, relax into the position, then try to twist a little further around. Hold for a count of 5, then relax forward. Do the extra twist 3 times. Then repeat the whole sequence using your other hand and leg.

Allow your head to turn naturally with your upper body

EASY ALTERNATIVE

Sit straight in a chair, cross one leg over the other and cross your forearms at shoulder height. Twist your head and upper body around to one side, then to the other to look behind you. Do this 5 times, then change legs, and repeat the sequence another 5 times.

The Pilates Roll

Weak abdominal muscles and incorrect posture are the main causes of an accentuated curve in the lumbar spine—lumbar lordosis. This can lead to back pain and even sciatica. The Pilates Roll helps prevent and treat such problems.

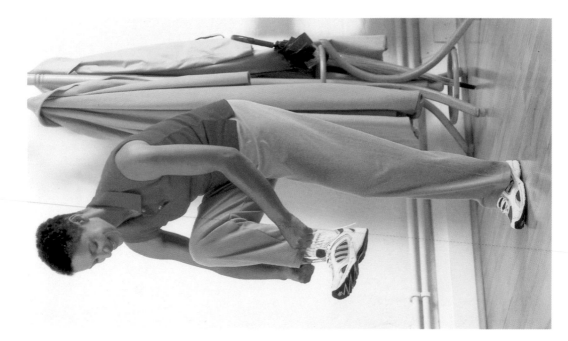

The Pilates Roll will help you with activities that involve using your stomach muscles to hold your body upright, such as tying your shoelaces while standing on one leg.

This Pilates exercise flattens the small of the back, and strengthens the straight abdominal muscles. It is important to keep these muscles strong as they counterbalance the muscles of the back, support the spine at its front, and keep the abdominal contents firmly in position.

Remember to keep your chin and stomach tucked in throughout this exercise, and to breathe deeply as you perform the movement. The roll should be performed on a suitably thick mat in order to cushion your spinous processes as you rock gently backward and forward.

PROGRESSION

Do the Main Exercise as before, but while balancing in Step 3, stretch your legs out in front of you, still slightly bent. Hold for a count of 5, and return to Step 3. Repeat this 5 times in total.

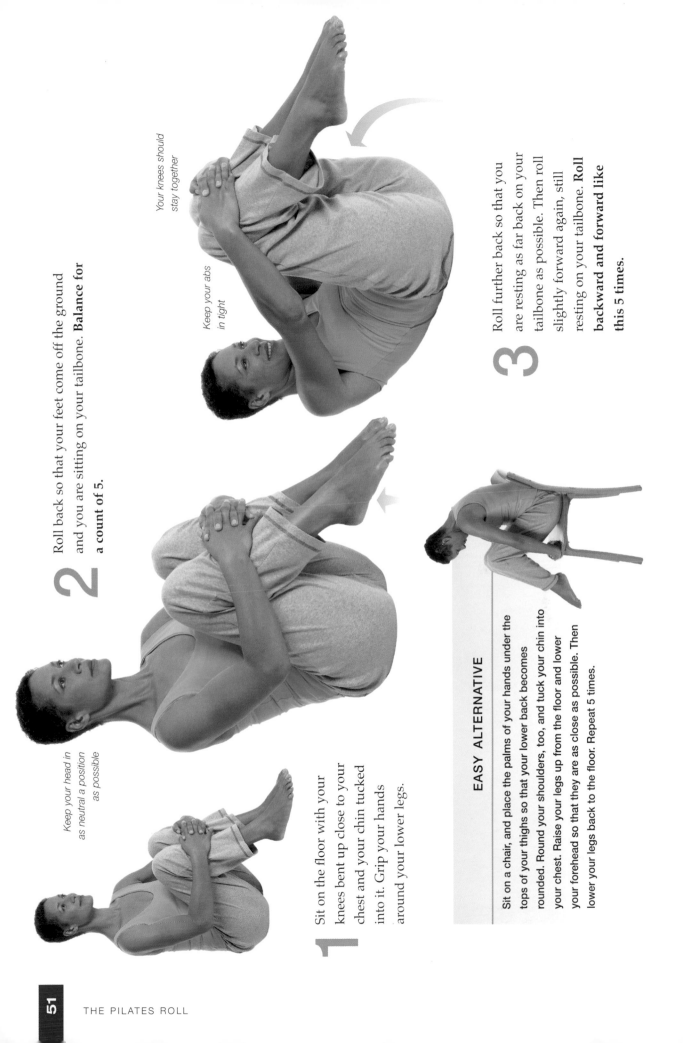

Your knees should stay together

Keep your abs in tight

2 Roll back so that your feet come off the ground and you are sitting on your tailbone. **Balance for a count of 5.**

3 Roll further back so that you are resting as far back on your tailbone as possible. Then roll slightly forward again, still resting on your tailbone. **Roll backward and forward like this 5 times.**

Keep your head in as neutral a position as possible

1 Sit on the floor with your knees bent up close to your chest and your chin tucked into it. Grip your hands around your lower legs.

EASY ALTERNATIVE

Sit on a chair, and place the palms of your hands under the tops of your thighs so that your lower back becomes rounded. Round your shoulders, too, and tuck your chin into your chest. Raise your legs up from the floor and lower your forehead so that they are as close as possible. Then lower your legs back to the floor. Repeat 5 times.

Shoulder Rolls

Many people who sit at a desk all day don't realize how much their shoulders hunch up and tighten, and their chests cave in. This compresses the vertebrae, which not only reduces breathing efficiency, but can also cause muscle spasms, tension headaches, and pain in the neck and upper chest. Shoulder Rolls will help prevent this.

PURPOSE

To improve breathing efficiency, and help prevent tension headaches by mobilizing the joints of the chest. This reduces the chance of discomfort in the neck, upper back, and shoulder muscles.

Is it right for me?

This exercise is suitable for people of all back types. If you have rounded shoulders, do the exercise as given. If you have a flat back, always complete the exercise on a forward roll rather than a backward one (see Step 3).

This exercise loosens the shoulders and neck, the shoulder blades, the joints between the ribs and the spine, and the joints between the ribs and the breastbone. It will therefore make you more flexible in your upper body movements, as well as allowing easier and more efficient breathing.

Shoulder Rolls also reduce tension in the muscles and ligaments, and encourage the intervertebral disks to absorb fluid, thus reducing wear and tear on the spine, and slowing down the onset of osteoarthritis. It's a good way of relieving tension quickly.

PROGRESSION

Simultaneously circle your arms 5 times, moving each arm in an opposite direction: one forward and the other backward. Repeat 5 times, starting each arm in the other direction to before. You'll need to be flexible and very co-ordinated for this movement. Make sure you finish by circling both arms backward to open out your rib cage.

Some people find the Shoulder Rolls Progression difficult to master because it requires a lot of coordination.

1 Sit with your lower back in a neutral position. Slowly circle both shoulders backward **5 times**. Then **repeat 5 times** in a forward direction.

Keep your feet flat on the floor

2 Circle your elbows instead of your shoulders. Slowly move them in a backward direction **5 times**. Then **repeat 5 times** in a forward direction.

Keep your head in a neutral position

Do not let your back arch

3 Complete the exercise by circling your arms backward **5 times**, in order to open out the chest, and stretch the neck muscles.

EASY ALTERNATIVE

If you don't have a stool or chair, you can do this whole sequence standing. Be careful, though, to keep the lower half of your body still, and to maintain the correct tilt of your pelvis. Your lower back must not be arched, otherwise it will take too much strain.

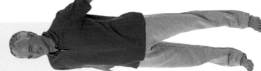

Chest Opener

A sedentary lifestyle means that the muscles of the chest and rib cage can become too tight. To compensate, the muscles of the upper back can become stretched and the shoulder blades may become immobile. This can lead to areas of tight, painful, knotted muscles. The Chest Opener will help prevent any such pain.

The Chest Opener Progression can be done anywhere and at any time. Try it during your lunch break to relieve tension.

PURPOSE

To counteract rounded shoulders by opening up the rib cage, loosening the costo-vertebral joints, mobilizing the thoracic spine, and strengthening the muscles of the chest.

Is it right for me?

This is suitable for people of all back types. It is especially useful for sedentary workers, and people with hunched shoulders, an exaggerated curve in the thoracic spine, or a pigeon chest.

This simple exercise opens up the chest. It stretches out the pectorals and strengthens the *trapezius* muscles. The movement of these muscles splays out the rib cage, stretching the ligaments and muscles that bind the ribs to the spine at the back and the sternum at the front.

This will make your breathing easier and more efficient, reduce tension, and mobilize the shoulder blades, making everyday upper body movements, like twisting, more comfortable.

PROGRESSION

Either sitting or standing, lift both arms straight in front of your body at shoulder height. Bend your elbows out, keeping your arms horizontal at shoulder height, and place one hand over the other. Pull your elbows out wide and back at shoulder height (see right), pushing your shoulder blades together. Repeat 5 times. Finish the exercise breathing in deeply with your arms in the pulled back position. Hold for a count of 10, then relax. Make sure that you do not let your shoulders hunch up during this exercise. Keep them in a relaxed position.

3 Open your arms out wide, keeping your elbows at shoulder height, and pushing your shoulder blades together. **Hold for a count of 10, then repeat the whole sequence 5 times.** Finish by breathing in deeply with your arms held open. **Hold for a count of 10**, then relax.

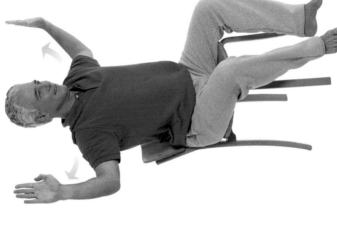

Relax your shoulders

Do not let your head drop forward

Your back should be straight

Do the same movement as in the Main Exercise but start with your elbows at waist level. Move them higher up the body with each repetition, until they reach the level of your head. Repeat 5 times in all.

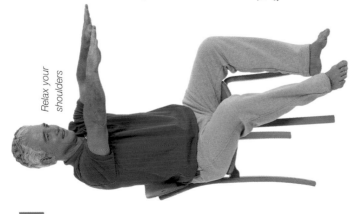

2 Raise your forearms so that they are at right angles to your upper arms. Move your arms together, so that the inner surfaces of your forearms and the palms of your hands touch each other. **Hold for a count of 10**, keeping your shoulders relaxed.

1 Take up the starting position by sitting tall in a chair, and lifting both arms up straight in front of your body at shoulder height. Make sure that your back is in a neutral position.

CHEST OPENER

Forearm Twist

Lack of exercise and incorrect posture can cause the joints between the vertebrae and their ligaments to tighten up. If this problem affects the upper back, breathing can be hampered. The Forearm Twist will help loosen these joints, and keep you flexible.

PURPOSE

To open the joints between the ribs and the thoracic vertebrae, and loosen the ligaments between them, in order to increase flexibility, and improve breathing.

Is it right for me?

This exercise is suitable for people of all back types. It is especially useful for people who have postural problems such as scoliosis of the spine (see also pages 84–85), or an overly flat, straight back.

The thoracic vertebrae, unlike the other vertebrae, are connected to the ribs by the costo-vertebral joints. This exercise stretches these costo-vertebral joints, and the ligaments around them, so that the rib cage remains flexible, and can expand to its full extent when you breathe in. It will therefore make everyday activities, such as stretching to the top shelf, or climbing stairs, easier for you to carry out.

The Forearm Twist is important as any tightness in the upper back area can inhibit the full movement of the ribs during breathing, limiting not only your flexibility but also your breathing efficiency. Practicing it regularly will steer you away from any such scenarios by keeping the upper back in full, working order.

PROGRESSION

During the last repetition of the exercise, unlock your hands, keeping one elbow over the other, and stretch each arm around toward the top of its opposite shoulder blade—as if you are hugging yourself. Hold for a count of 10. Relax, then repeat 4 times, stretching further around each time if possible.

If doing the Forearm Twist Progression on a chair, you should aim for your hands to reach the back of the chair, rather than opposing shoulder blades.

3 Relax your shoulders, and push your arms up as far as possible. **Hold for a count of 10. Repeat 5 times, then repeat the exercise** with the opposite elbow on top.

EASY ALTERNATIVE

If you can't manage to twist your arms enough for the Main Exercise, stretch both arms straight in front at shoulder height instead. Link your hands, and push them forward as far as you can. This exercise is even more beneficial if you use wrist weights.

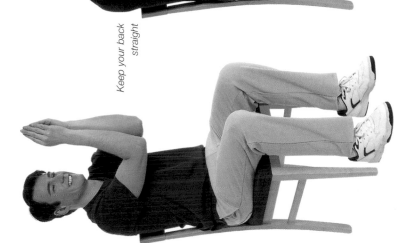

Keep your feet flat on the floor

Try not to hunch up your shoulders when doing this

Keep your back straight

2 Put one elbow over the other, and gently twist your forearms so that the fingers of your top hand can grasp the fingers of your bottom hand.

1 Sit with your back in a neutral position, and raise your arms in front of you. Bend your elbows so that your forearms are at right angles to your upper arms, and your forearms and palms are touching.

Side Bends

If one group of back muscles stays tight for too long, its opposing group becomes overstretched and weak. This can twist the spine to the side, or distort its natural curves, compressing the vertebrae and increasing wear and tear on disks. Side Bends to alternate sides will help prevent any such imbalance and resulting discomfort.

PURPOSE

To increase flexibility, and to reduce wear and tear on the spine by stretching the muscles and ligaments of the back and rib cage, and by opening up the sides of the vertebrae.

Is it right for me?

This exercise is suitable for people of all back types. It is especially useful for people with a sideways curve in the spine (scoliosis), or those with a flat back.

This exercise will stretch the muscles of the back and rib cage, easing the strain on the spine. Side Bends also open up the right and left sides of the vertebrae alternately, helping maintain muscular balance, and encouraging the intervertebral disks to absorb fluid. This prevents the disks grinding on one another, thus avoiding unnecessary wear and tear on the spine, and helping to slow down the onset of osteoarthritis.

Bad habits can be the source of problems with muscular imbalance. For example, if you regularly carry a heavy bag with a shoulder strap, your spine may develop a curve to the side on which you most often carry it; or if you stand overly straight, your tightened muscles may distort your spine's natural curves. When doing Side Bends to ease these problems, always stretch the side that you feel is the tightest first.

CAUTION

Only bend to the side during this exercise. Any forward, backward, or rotational movement can decrease the value of the exercise by putting uneven pressure on the disks.

PROGRESSION

Intertwine your fingers, turn your palms up, and stretch them as far as possible above your head. Then do the Main Exercise as before.

Make sure you keep your intertwined hands above your head when doing the Side Bends Progression. Do not let them go behind your head as this may cause you to arch your back.

SIDE BENDS

Do the movement as in the Main Exercise but slide your lower hand down the side of the body as far as possible, instead of keeping it on your waist.

Do not lean forward or backward during the movement

Keep your knees slightly bent

3 Bend more at the waist to increase the stretch. **Do this exercise on the other side, then repeat the whole sequence 5 times.**

Remember to breathe deeply as you do the exercise

Relax both your shoulders

Keep your feet flat on the floor

1 Stand with your feet shoulder-width apart, your knees slightly bent, and your hands resting loosely on your waist. Keep your head still, looking forward, and your weight evenly balanced.

2 Stretch one hand up and over your head as you gently lean to the side. Tilt your head in the same direction as you are moving your hand and body. **Hold for a count of 10.**

Pec Stretch

Having hunched shoulders can start to feel natural with time. But you should not allow yourself to fall into this trap. Instead, constantly strive to acquire better posture as it not only reduces your chances of getting back problems, but also gives you a sense of improved well-being. The Pec Stretch will help you achieve this goal.

PURPOSE

To expand the chest, mobilize the joints between the ribs and the breastbone, and counteract the negative effects of a slouched posture.

Is it right for me?

This exercise is suitable for people of all back types. It is especially useful for people with hunched shoulders, and those who lead a sedentary lifestyle.

This exercise counters the harmful effects of hunched shoulders by opening up the chest, mobilizing the rib joints at the breastbone, and strengthening the large muscles of the back. This means you can enjoy the benefits of improved posture, which often brings with it improved self-confidence, as well as a stronger, healthier back.

Having hunched shoulders throws your center of gravity forward. This stretches the postural muscles of the back, disrupting the alignment of the spinal joints, and causing the pectoral muscles of the chest to tighten in compensation. By regularly practicing the Pec Stretch you will help prevent your back adapting to this habitual bad posture.

PROGRESSION

Hold on to both sides of a doorway with your arms behind you at approximately chest height.

Straighten your arms, and lean forward so that your body weight increases the stretch across your upper chest. Keep your elbows slightly bent throughout.

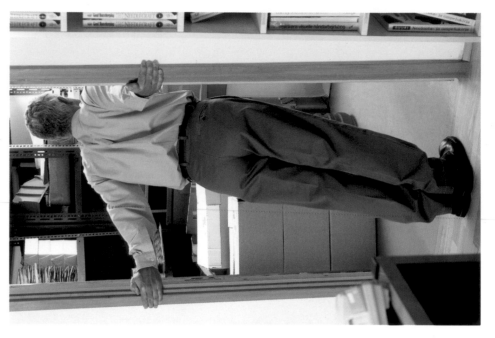

The Pec Stretch Progression can be carried out wherever there is a stable doorway free to use as support. Only lean as far forward as you feel is safe and comfortable.

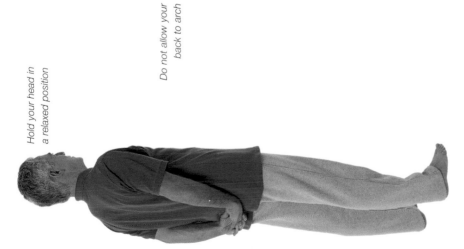

EASY ALTERNATIVE

Hold a towel horizontally behind your back, grasping it at both ends. Raise the towel slowly upward over your head (bending one elbow up to do so), down to waist height, and then right back again. Finish with your hands behind your back.

Make sure your pelvis is "tucked"

Relax your shoulders

Do not allow your back to arch

Hold your head in a relaxed position

1 Stand with your feet hip-width apart, and interlace your fingers behind your back with your palms facing up. Keep your chin tucked in so that you do not lean forward, reducing the stretch.

2 Slowly straighten your arms while turning your elbows in toward your spine. Keep your back in a neutral position, and your shoulders relaxed. **Hold the stretch for a count of 10.**

3 Pull in your abdominal muscles to avoid arching your back, and lift your arms up as far as possible behind you. **Hold for a count of 10,** then lower and relax. **Repeat the sequence 5 times.**

Thoracic Stretch

One of the problems for people with rounded shoulders is that the vertebrae on the inner side of their spines become compressed. This increases wear and tear on both the spine and its disks, and compresses the joints, causing inflammation and pain. The Thoracic Stretch will help counteract any such problems.

PURPOSE

To improve posture and flexibility by opening out the inner surfaces of the vertebrae, and stretching the thoracic spine and its muscles and ligaments.

Is it right for me?

This exercise is suitable for people of all back types. It is especially useful for those with rounded shoulders. If you have a shoulder problem, such as frozen shoulder or osteoarthritis, the Easy Alternative form of the exercise is better.

This exercise stretches the joints, ligaments, and muscles on the inner surface of the spine. It also opens the shoulders out. This will make it easier for you to carry out everyday movements like bending and turning, such as when lifting shopping bags out of the trunk of the car, or weeding in the yard.

The Thoracic Stretch is not an easy exercise to do correctly as there is a tendency to tighten the muscles between your arms and your shoulder blades during the movement. If you feel the pull mainly in your shoulders, make a conscious effort to relax your upper body. If it still isn't comfortable, try the Easy Alternative instead.

You can practice the Thoracic Stretch Progression any time you have both a spare moment and a clear area of wall. Try to keep your knees facing forward as much as you can.

PROGRESSION

Stand with your back a forearm-length away from a wall. Twist your body and arms slowly around to one side until you can put your hands flat on the wall. Hold the stretch for a count of 30, then repeat on the other side.

CAUTION

Take care when doing the Progression exercise if you have any knee problems, as it places some strain on the knees.

1 Place your hands and feet shoulder-width apart, keeping your knees slightly bent. Then bend over to lean on a sturdy support, like a chair, table, or the back of a chair. Allow your back to arch as much as is comfortable. Relax into the position, and **hold for a count of 30**. Your bottom will stick out as you do this.

Your head should be the last part of your body to return to the starting position

Stand with your feet hip-width apart, and your back in a neutral position. Hollow your back as much as you can by pulling your shoulders and bottom back. Hold for a count of 10. Bring your back into a neutral position. Repeat 5 times. Then reverse the stretch by rounding your back as much as you can. Hold for a count of 10. Repeat 5 times.

Keep your knees slightly bent

2 Gradually return to standing by bending your knees further, and rounding your back as you rise. You can change the height of your support and therefore your hands to feel the stretch in different areas of the back. **Repeat the exercise 3 times.**

The Sitting Plough

If your upper back is too flat and straight, your ribs will join the vertebrae at an incorrect angle. This puts strain on the joints, can affect your breathing, and can cause a stitch-like pain around the chest wall, and beneath the shoulder blades. The Sitting Plough will steer you away from any such trouble.

PURPOSE

To stretch the vertebrae and ribs of the upper back, stretch the two ligaments that run down each side of the spine, and stretch the intervertebral ligaments in order to maintain and restore the natural curve of the upper spine.

Is it right for me?

This exercise is suitable for people of all back types.

This exercise is an adaptation of the yoga plough exercise, which is given as a Progression. However, we offer a sitting adaptation as the Main Exercise because few people can get into the correct yoga position without considerable practice. It is important to breathe deeply during this movement, and not to force your neck unnecessarily forward.

PROGRESSION

Lie on your back, and bend your knees to your chest, leaving your arms straight on the floor. Straighten your legs as you pull your back up off the mat, then bring your legs as close to the floor as possible behind your head, so that your toes reach toward the floor. Hold this position for as long as is comfortable. Then gradually roll out of it, and relax.

You can place your legs on a chair or stool behind your head if your feet can not yet reach the floor when doing the Sitting Plough Progression.

CAUTION

People with neck problems and those over 60 should consult a doctor before attempting this exercise. There is a risk that blood flow to the brain could be interrupted during the exercise if arteries supplying the head have already been pinched by osteoarthritis or inflammation (arteritis).

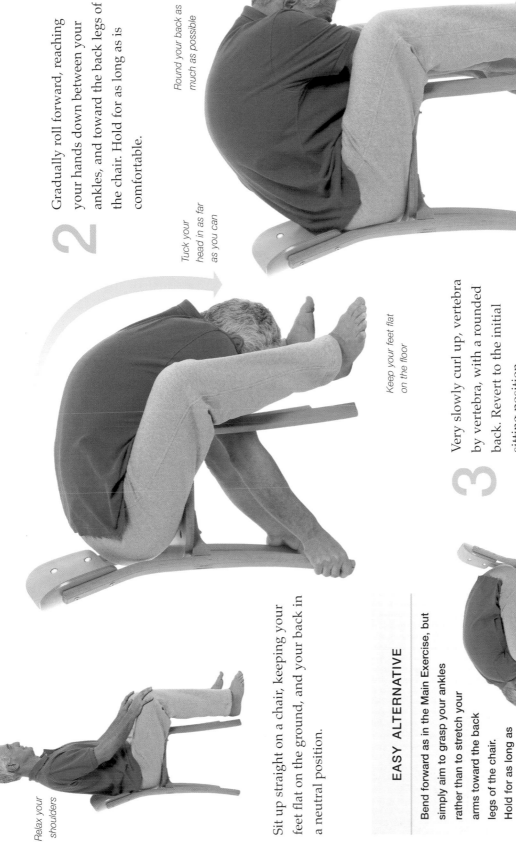

2 Gradually roll forward, reaching your hands down between your ankles, and toward the back legs of the chair. Hold for as long as is comfortable.

Round your back as much as possible

Tuck your head in as far as you can

Keep your feet flat on the floor

3 Very slowly curl up, vertebra by vertebra, with a rounded back. Revert to the initial sitting position.

1 Sit up straight on a chair, keeping your feet flat on the ground, and your back in a neutral position.

EASY ALTERNATIVE

Bend forward as in the Main Exercise, but simply aim to grasp your ankles rather than to stretch your arms toward the back legs of the chair. Hold for as long as is comfortable, then curl up.

Relax your shoulders

Back Extender

Your lower back muscles provide your back with stability, mobility, and strength. If these muscles are weak, many of your daily movements would be greatly restricted. The Back Extender will help keep the lower back muscles strong, flexible, and fully capable of their job.

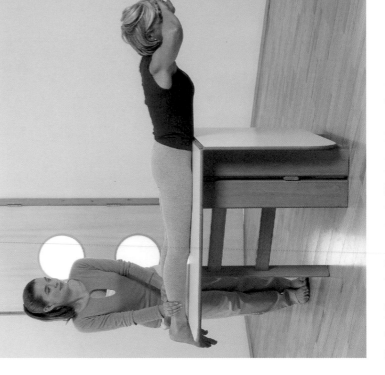

This exercise works all the muscle groups that support the back and spine except for the very small ones that allow rotation.

It is very important that all movements in the Back Extender are performed with complete muscular control. If you allow yourself to flop down, you could pull or tear small muscles. This could make neighboring muscles go into spasm, in order to prevent any more movement in the area, which might cause more damage. Move slowly to avoid hurting yourself.

PURPOSE

To strengthen the muscles of the lower back, increasing support for the spine, and to open up the side of the spine nearest the stomach.

Is it right for me?

This exercise is suitable for people of all back types. If you have weak back muscles, do not to lift up too far. It is important that the downward movement is under complete control.

PROGRESSION

Lie on your stomach across a stable surface with your hips at its edge (see right). Ask a helper to hold your legs down. Start with your body hanging down off the surface, and your hands crossed over your forehead. Pull in your stomach muscles to lift your body up as far as is comfortable. Keep your back straight, and do not lift too far, as you must be able to control the downward movement. Hold for a count of 3, then lower. Repeat 5 times.

The Back Extender Progression is difficult, but it is an effective way to work out the back muscles—tightening them as you move up, and releasing them as you gradually move down.

CAUTION

It is important to do the Essential Follow-up immediately after the Back Extender, as well as after the Back Extender Progression, in order to release any tension and pressure that may have built up in the lower back.

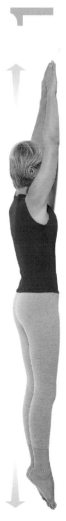

1 Lie on your stomach with your hands straight out above your head. Stretch out, elongating your body as much as possible. **Hold for a count of 10**, then relax. **Repeat 3 times.**

Do not let the lifting leg twist

2 Rest your head on your hands, and lift one leg slowly off the floor, taking care not to let it twist. Your leg should only lift a short way from the floor. **Hold for a count of 10**, then lower slowly. **Do this 5 times, then repeat with your other leg.**

Keep your neck in a neutral position

Keep your legs firmly on the floor

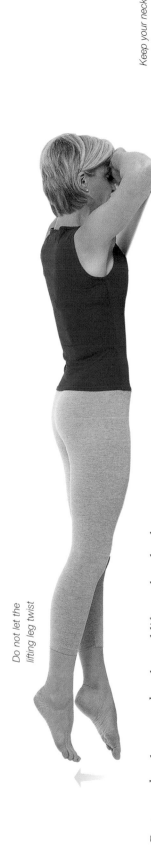

3 Relax your legs, and place your forehead on your hands. Raise your back, shoulders, and head a little off the floor, being careful not to arch your neck. **Hold for a count of 3,** then lower slowly. **Repeat 5 times.**

ESSENTIAL FOLLOW-UP

Do this to release any pressure in your spine after the Back Extender. Roll slowly onto your back. Bend your knees, leaving your feet flat on the floor, and your knees hip-width apart. Lift one knee toward your chest, pulling it in with your hands, then lower it. Do this 3 times, then repeat with your other knee.

Cross Abs

A lot of people have relatively weak abdominal muscles, which is unfortunate as abdominal weakness is responsible for the majority of back problems. We have two main sets of abdominal muscles—primary and oblique. The Cross Abs exercise will help you strengthen both.

PURPOSE

To work and strengthen the abdominal muscles, which increase support for the spine and act as a counterbalance to the back muscles.

Is it right for me?

This exercise is suitable for people of all back types. It is especially useful for those with weak abdominal muscles, or a hollow back.

CAUTION

It is important not to put any strain on your neck when lifting and lowering your head. Do not let it fall too far back, or tuck it too far into your chest. Keep it in a neutral position.

This exercise works on strengthening the abdominal muscles so that they can act as an effective counterbalance to the back muscles.

Our primary abdominal muscles bend the spine forward, with the support of two groups of oblique abdominals: internal and external. The internal group moves the hip diagonally toward the opposite shoulder, while the external obliques move the shoulder diagonally toward the opposite hip.

The Cross Abs Progression works both these sets of oblique abdominal muscles.

PROGRESSION

Do the Main Exercise as before but now raise each knee toward the opposite arm, while raising each arm toward the opposite knee.

Make sure you keep your stomach muscles tightly pulled in as you do the Cross Abs Progression, and remember to keep breathing deeply.

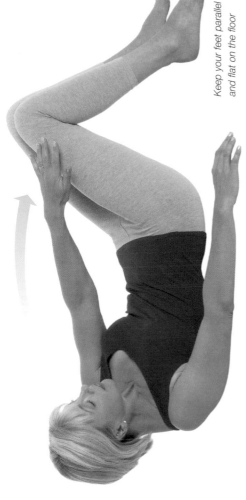

Your knees are hip-width apart

Keep your feet parallel and flat on the floor

1 Lie on your back with your knees bent and hip-width apart, and your feet flat on the floor. Tighten your stomach muscles so that you are pushing the small of your back into the mat.

2 Lift one hand toward the opposite knee, smoothly curling your back up, and raising your shoulder off the mat as you do so. Only lift a short way at first as the movement needs to be under control. **Hold for a count of 10, then lower slowly. Repeat 5 times.**

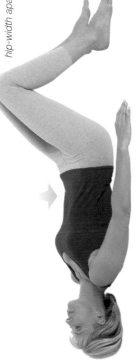

Keep your neck in a comfortable position

3 **Repeat the whole exercise to the other side.** Do not forget to breathe as you carry out the movements. It helps to breathe deeply—out on the way up, and in on the way down.

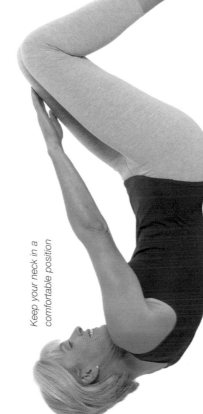

EASY ALTERNATIVE

Stand with your legs hip-width apart, and reach one hand down toward the opposite foot. Keep your back rounded, and allow the non-reaching arm to swing behind your body. Hold for a count of 10, then rise slowly to standing. Do this 5 times, then repeat to the other side.

LOWER BACK

Pelvic Lifts

Weakness in the buttock muscles often leads to poor posture, especially an accentuated hollow back and slouched shoulders. Pelvic Lifts will help you strengthen these muscles, and improve your posture.

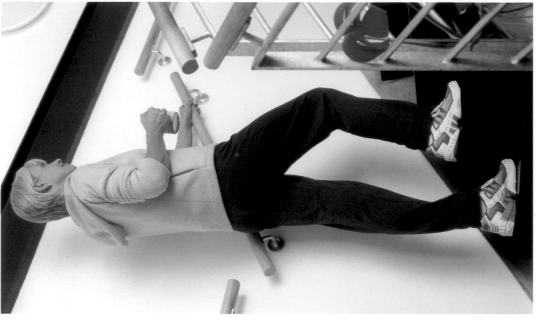

PURPOSE

To strengthen the thigh and buttock muscles, to learn to release the spine in a controlled way, and to spot any areas of weakness in your back.

Is it right for me?

This exercise is suitable for people of all back types. It is especially useful for those who have a hollow back.

This exercise strengthens the buttock muscles—the *glutei*. These are important because they stabilize the hip joints and lower back, and prevent the lower spine from bending forward when you walk or run.

The spine is constructed of a number of small bones—vertebrae—each of which is capable of small but significant movements. When these movements are isolated as you lower your pelvis, vertebra by vertebra, to the ground during Pelvic Lifts, you will be able to identify if any area is stiff, painful, or in need of extra attention.

PROGRESSION

Do the Main Exercise as before but turn each hip up and forward alternately before lowering your pelvis when in the raised position. Do this by first squeezing the muscles of one buttock, then those of the other buttock.

Work out while you walk by tucking your pelvis in when climbing up stairs. This way you are integrating Pelvic Lifts—and their benefits—into your everyday life.

1 Lie on your back with your knees bent and hip-width apart, and your feet flat on the floor. Tighten your stomach muscles so that you are pushing the small of your back into the mat.

Your knees are hip-width apart

2 Lift your buttocks off the ground so that your body forms a straight line from your shoulders to your knees. In this position, squeeze your buttock muscles tightly. **Hold for a count of 10.**

Lower down to the floor gradually

3 Relax your buttocks, and lower your body a little. Again raise into the full pelvic lift, squeeze the buttocks, and **hold for a count of 10.** Then slowly lower your body, vertebra by vertebra, to the mat. **Repeat the whole sequence 5 times.**

Keep your head in neutral position

EASY ALTERNATIVE

Sit on the floor with your legs straight out in front of you, and your arms stretched forward for balance. Now "walk" forward on your bottom for 6 paces, then back for 6. Repeat 3 times. Make sure that the opposite arm and leg always move together, just as when walking normally.

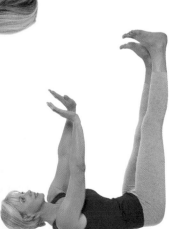

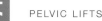

Side Leg Raises

A hip joint that is not regularly put through its full range of movement can easily become stiff, which can increase pressure on the lower spine. Side Leg Raises will help prevent stiffness and pressure by stretching the hips through a much greater range of movement than they are used to in everyday activities.

PURPOSE

To strengthen the thigh and buttock muscles in order to stabilize the hip and pelvis, and add extra support to the lower back.

Is it right for me?

This exercise is suitable for people of all back types.

This exercise will help you maintain flexibility, and prevent stiffness in your hips. Side Leg Raises also increase support for your lower back.

It is interesting to note that stiffness and osteoarthritis of the hip is far more common in the West than in the East, where many people sit cross-legged, or in the more advanced Lotus position—the same as cross-legged but with each foot resting on the opposite knee. Such positions stretch the abductor and adductor muscles at the side of the thigh and pelvis, keeping them flexible. Performing Side Leg Raises works these same muscles, rather than stretching them.

PROGRESSION

Do the Main Exercise as before but now rotate the hip of your upper leg as you raise it so that your toes are pointing straight up. Be careful not to hollow your lower back. Then turn your foot in on each lowering of the leg so that your toes point to the floor.

Try to get into the habit of sitting cross-legged on the floor when you are relaxing as this stretches out your leg muscles.

EASY ALTERNATIVE

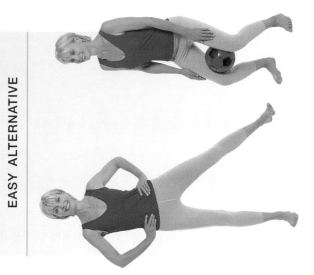

Stand with your feet shoulder-width apart. Swing one leg straight out to the side, hold for a count of 3 at the furthest point, and lower slowly. Do this 5 times, then repeat the sequence with your other leg. Next, place a ball between your knees, and squeeze it by pushing your knees together for a count of 10, without allowing your toes to turn inward. Finish by relaxing into a normal standing position.

Relax your head

Keep this hand on the floor for balance

1 Lie on one side with your bottom leg bent, and your head resting on your bottom arm. Make sure you don't let yourself roll forward or backward at any point during this exercise. Raise your top leg, being careful not to twist it. **Hold for a count of 5,** then slowly lower it. **Repeat 5 times.**

Keep your abs pulled in tight

2 Bend your top leg, and drop it over onto the floor in front of you. Straighten your bottom leg, then lift it up. It will not lift far off the ground. **Hold for a count of 5,** then lower. **Repeat 5 times.** Then turn onto your other side, and **repeat the whole sequence.**

Sitting Hip Roll

If your back becomes stiff and rigid through lack of exercise, spine rotation is often the first movement to suffer. Even turning and lifting objects can seem difficult. The Sitting Hip Roll will help you strengthen the ligaments and muscles of your back to prevent this situation.

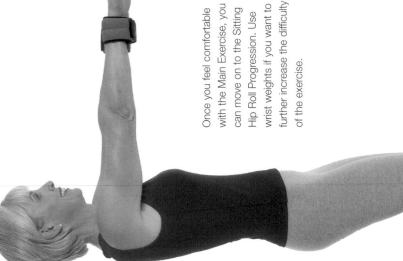

This exercise increases the flexibility of the thoracic and lumbar spine by stretching the small muscles and ligaments, and loosening the vertebral joints.

While the ligaments and muscles of the back support it well during forward-bending, side-bending, and arching, they offer much less support during rotation. The Sitting Hip Roll will help you strengthen them so that your ability to rotate in everyday movements does not become hampered. An inability to rotate is not only inconvenient, but also can cause the spine to stiffen up, intervertebral disks to shrink, and spinal joints to be pushed together, resulting in osteoarthritis. The Sitting Hip Roll is therefore very beneficial.

PROGRESSION

Do the Main Exercise as below but alter the central position. Instead of brushing your buttocks on your heels as you move from side to side, lift the buttocks entirely, so that you are kneeling upright between each side-sit, with your upper legs in line with your straight back.
Use your arms for balance.

Once you feel comfortable with the Main Exercise, you can move on to the Sitting Hip Roll Progression. Use wrist weights if you want to further increase the difficulty of the exercise.

PURPOSE

To increase the flexibility of the lower spine in rotation, and to strengthen the stomach and back muscles.

Is it right for me?

This exercise is suitable for people of all back types. If your back is stiff and inflexible, you should start with the Easy Alternative and build up from it.

CAUTION

If you have osteoarthritis of the spine or problems with balance, check with your doctor or physical therapist before trying this exercise.

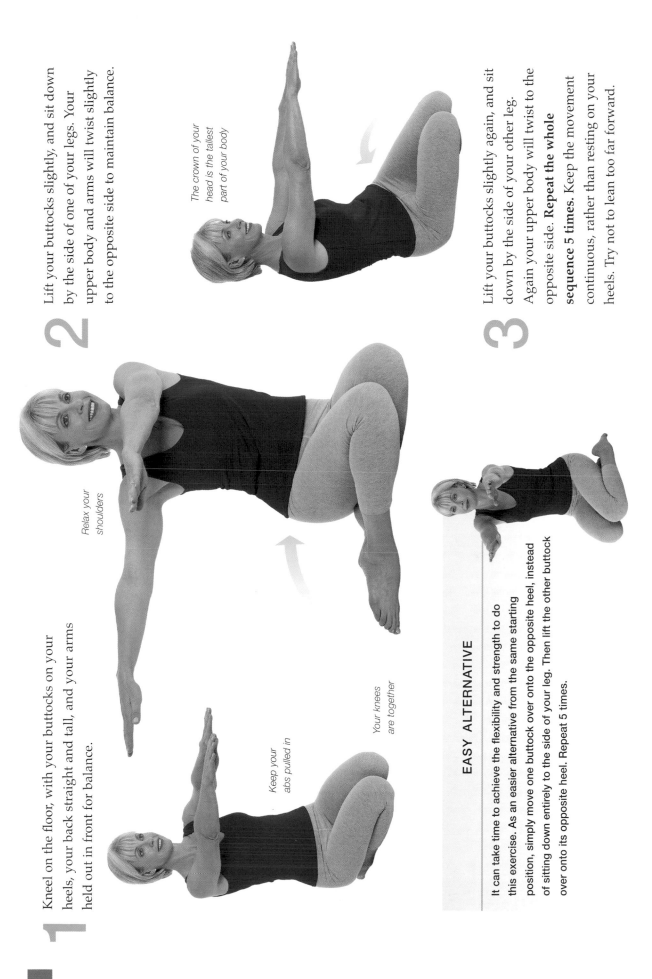

1 Kneel on the floor, with your buttocks on your heels, your back straight and tall, and your arms held out in front for balance.

Relax your shoulders

Keep your abs pulled in

Your knees are together

2 Lift your buttocks slightly, and sit down by the side of one of your legs. Your upper body and arms will twist slightly to the opposite side to maintain balance.

The crown of your head is the tallest part of your body

3 Lift your buttocks slightly again, and sit down by the side of your other leg. Again your upper body will twist to the opposite side. **Repeat the whole sequence 5 times.** Keep the movement continuous, rather than resting on your heels. Try not to lean too far forward.

EASY ALTERNATIVE

It can take time to achieve the flexibility and strength to do this exercise. As an easier alternative from the same starting position, simply move one buttock over onto the opposite heel, instead of sitting down entirely to the side of your leg. Then lift the other buttock over onto its opposite heel. Repeat 5 times.

The Saw

A Pilates exercise, The Saw emphasizes the importance of what is known as the "powerhouse"—the muscles of the lower back, abdomen, and thighs—in maintaining correct posture and balance, both of which are essential for a healthy back.

PURPOSE

To stretch and mobilize the lower back and hamstrings, to increase your ability to maintain tension in the stomach muscles, and to promote awareness of controlled breathing.

Is it right for me?

This exercise is suitable for people of all back types. It is especially useful for those who have a hollow back or weak abdominal muscles.

As with all Pilates exercises, The Saw is designed to increase the body's suppleness and grace in everyday activities. It combines controlled breathing with stretching the lower back, waist, and hips. It is important that you keep your stomach muscles tight throughout the movement.

This exercise should be performed in a controlled manner, while you concentrate on the correct position of your body. You will need a small, rolled-up towel for the Easy Alternative of this exercise.

chest, leaving your arms by your sides on the mat for balance. Pull in your stomach muscles, and breathe in as you slowly roll back so that your hips reach either side of your face, your feet and lower legs reach toward the floor, and you are balancing on your shoulder blades. Keep your knees bent, and use your arms to support your lower back on the way up if necessary. Hold for as long as is comfortable. Then breathe out as you tighten your stomach muscles to roll slowly and gradually back into a lying position.

PROGRESSION

Lie on your back with your knees bent, and bring them up to your

The Saw Progression is a difficult one to master. Only attempt it if you have become very confident with the Main Exercise.

THE SAW

1 Sit with your legs stretched out in a V in front of you, keeping your knees flat on the floor, and your toes pulled up. Raise your arms straight out to the sides at shoulder height, and tighten your stomach muscles.

Pull in your abs

EASY ALTERNATIVE

**Tight hamstrings may make it difficult to do this at first. Instead of braving any pain or discomfort, try placing a small, rolled-up towel beneath each of your knees. This reduces the stretch on the muscle, yet still allows you to perform the movement correctly.
Then perform the exercise as explained in the Main Exercise Steps.**

2 Breathe in, and then out deeply as you round your back and reach one hand down toward the little toe of the opposite foot. Allow your other arm to swing behind you as you do this. **Hold for a count of 10.** Breathe in as you roll up, vertebra by vertebra, to the starting position.

Round your back

Try to keep your knees on the floor

Don't allow your head to jut forward

3 **Do this on the other side, then repeat the whole sequence 3 times.** Keep your head in a neutral position throughout the exercise to avoid straining your neck.

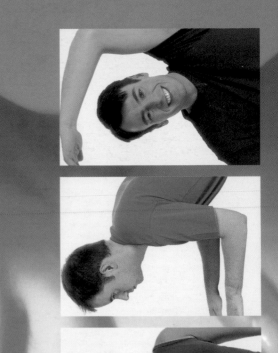
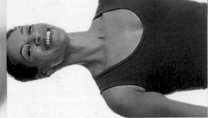
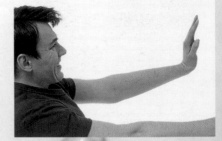

Problem Backs

Four of the most common back problems are discussed here: sciatica, osteoarthritis, scoliosis, and osteoporosis. Bear in mind, however, that osteoarthritis and osteoporosis often affect areas other than the back.

In this section you will find information on each of the conditions, and ways of trying to alleviate symptoms. There is an initial gentle exercise recommended for each, which is specially designed to be safe and comfortable to perform, as well as to relieve any pain you feel. Once you are confident and at ease with this exercise, move onto the mini-program of exercises provided for each before trying any other exercises in the book.

If you suffer from any back disorder, whether discussed in this section or not, it is important to:

- consult your doctor or physical therapist before beginning any exercise program;
- read the introduction to each exercise carefully to make sure it is suitable for you;
- pay particular attention to Effective Exercise Techniques (page 13).

Sciatica

The pain caused by sciatica can feel as if it comes from the whole of the sciatic nerve's course, from the lower back to the foot, although the condition is the result of problems in the back. These exercises can help prevent and ease the pain.

Pain caused by a pinched sciatic nerve starts in the lower back, and can spread right down the legs.

This problem arises when an inflamed facet joint, intervertebral disk, or a bony spur pinches the sciatic nerve as it leaves the spine. Factors such as poor lifting technique, or sudden strenuous movement can trigger the acute bursts of sharp pain associated with sciatica.

The exercise below is designed to relieve the cause of the pinching, and reduce the stretch of the sciatic nerve affected. It also promotes relaxation of the tiny muscles that connect the vertebrae and facet joints, which go into immediate spasm on the onset of the pain of sciatica, increasing the pinching effect. Try the exercise five times a day during an attack, and use it as part of your normal back routine at other times.

PREVENTION AND TREATMENT

- Always be aware of your posture.
- Exercise regularly, and avoid sudden bursts of unaccustomed, strenuous exercise.
- Learn how to lift objects correctly (see page 20).
- Practice Pelvic Tilts frequently (see pages 36–37).

PURPOSE

The exercise below is to help reduce inflammation, and open up the spine so that the intervertebral disks can absorb fluid, thus reducing any bulging, and helping keep the bones of the facet joints apart and mobile.

Is it right for me?

This exercise is suitable for people of all back types. People with hollow backs should omit Step 2, which hollows the back further. Women in advanced stages of pregnancy should not do this exercise.

CAUTION

If you have been in an accident and can feel the sharp pain associated with sciatica, do not move. Ask for medical help in case part of the spine is pressing on the spinal cord.

1 Lie flat on your stomach with your arms by your sides, and your head turned to the side that hurts the least. Take a deep breath in, then relax completely as you exhale. Relax fully to reduce muscle spasms, and to allow the spine to realign itself. Keep breathing deeply in this position, relaxing into the pain. **Hold for 5 minutes.**

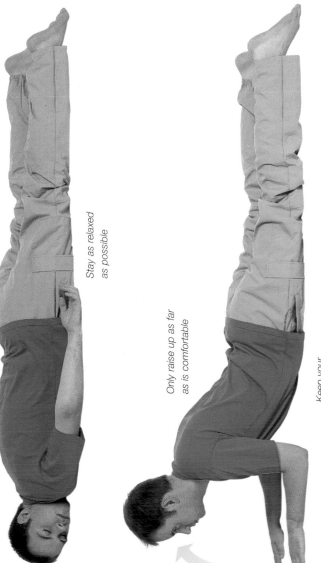

Stay as relaxed as possible

Only raise up as far as is comfortable

Keep your abs tight

2 Raise yourself up onto your elbows so that they are directly under your shoulders, with your hands pointed forward. Relax completely. **Hold for up to 5 minutes.** Return to the starting position, and breathe naturally.

MINI-PROGRAM

The exercise above is the most suitable isolated one to help you deal with ongoing pain. When the pain no longer runs down the leg but is centralized in the small of the back, move on to other exercises to create a mini-program that will help reduce pressure on the lower back. Start with:

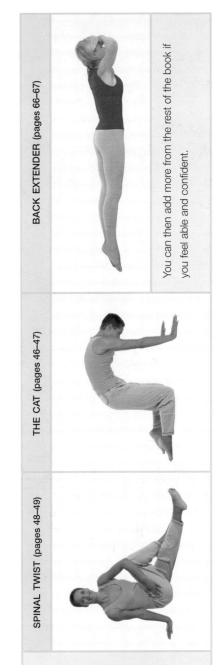

SPINAL TWIST (pages 48–49)

THE CAT (pages 46–47)

BACK EXTENDER (pages 66–67)

You can then add more from the rest of the book if you feel able and confident.

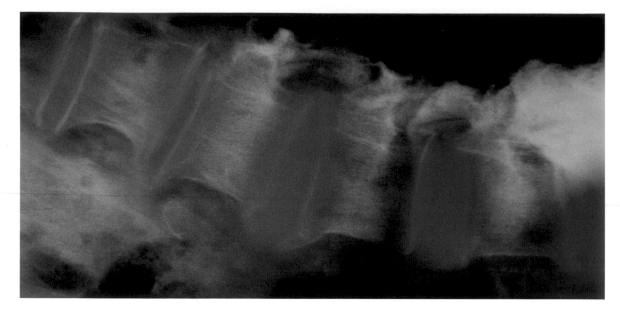

Osteoarthritis

This degenerative condition is a natural part of ageing, although it occurs occasionally in the young as a result of an injury or deformity. It mainly affects the cartilage and bone of weight-bearing joints. Certain exercises will help slow down the onset of this disorder.

Over the years, the layers of tough, flexible cartilage that line the joints become worn, thin, and brittle until the ends of the bones start to grind on each other. The cartilage also hardens, and produces bony spurs at the joint edges, which limit joint movement and can press on spinal nerve roots, resulting in stiffness and pain.

Some osteoarthritis is inevitable, but its onset can be slowed down by correct posture (see pages 8, 18, and 20), a moderate amount of suitable exercise, a healthy diet, and a good lifting technique (see page 20).

PREVENTION AND TREATMENT

- Concentrate on exercises to increase flexibility.
- Be aware of your posture, especially when sitting, as this creates more pressure on the spine than standing.
- Learn how to lift and carry objects correctly.
- Watch your weight (see page 93 for advice)—excess weight creates extra downward pressure on the spine.

This X ray of an osteoarthritic lower spine shows how the cartilage (red) has worn away, allowing the vertebrae (yellow) to rub on each other at the back of the spine (bottom right). This would cause great discomfort.

PURPOSE

The exercise below aims to move the joints of the spine through their full range of movement to lubricate the cartilage, and limit wear and tear on the joints.

Is it right for me?

This exercise is suitable for people of all back types. It will help prevent long-term discomfort, ease stiffness, and maintain joint movement in those who already suffer from osteoarthritis to some degree.

CAUTION

If you already suffer from osteoarthritis and stiffness, start with the Easy Alternative of each exercise in order to give yourself a gentle introduction to the Main Exercise Steps.

OSTEOARTHRITIS

Relax your head and neck

Keep your head tucked in

1 Lie on your side with your arms stretched out above your head, and your legs stretched out straight.

2 Curl up into a ball, bringing your head and knees into your chest, and wrap your arms around your legs. Feel the stretch down your spine, and **hold for a count of 10.**

Keep your abs tight

Keep your legs together

3 Uncurl, and stretch out so that your back forms a bow. **Hold for a count of 10. Repeat the whole sequence 5 times.** Then roll over onto your other side, and **repeat the exercise 5 times.**

MINI-PROGRAM

The exercise on the left is the most suitable isolated one for you to perform. Once you are comfortable with it, you should aim to add more exercises to create a mini-program. Start with:

PELVIC TILTS (pages 36–37)

THE CAT (pages 46–47)

BACK EXTENDER (pages 66–67)

You can then add more from the rest of the book if you feel able and confident.

Scoliosis

More common than you may think, scoliosis affects approximately two per cent of the population. If your spine forms a "C" or "S" shape when viewed from the back, you have scoliosis—a sideways bend in the spine. Certain exercises can help with this problem.

The red "S" bend shows the shape that the spine of a scoliosis sufferer might be. Notice how distorted it is in comparison to the man's healthy, straight spine beneath.

A minor bend in the spine is not uncommon, and is usually caused either by a small difference in the length of the legs, or by overuse of the muscles on one side of the spine, and underuse on the other side.

The muscles on the side of the spine that is underused become weak—forming the inside of the curve. The overworked muscles on the other side become shortened and stiff—forming the outside of the curve. Eventually, it becomes increasingly hard to straighten the spine, as the ligaments adapt to the habitual posture. These unequal stresses on the spine cause pain and muscular aches, and may also lead to osteoarthritis.

PREVENTION AND TREATMENT

- Seek your doctor's advice.
- Stretch out the overworked muscles, and strengthen those on the opposing side.
- Use alternate hands when carrying heavy objects, or carry an equal load in each hand.

PURPOSE

The exercise below aims to straighten any problematic curves in the spine by strengthening and stretching the muscles and ligaments in the back.

Is it right for me?

This is an excellent exercise for anyone with mild scoliosis of the spine. However, in more severe cases specialist exercises, orthopedic braces, and sometimes even surgery may be needed.

CAUTION

People who suffer from scoliosis may also develop sciatica. See pages 80–81 for advice on how to deal with this.

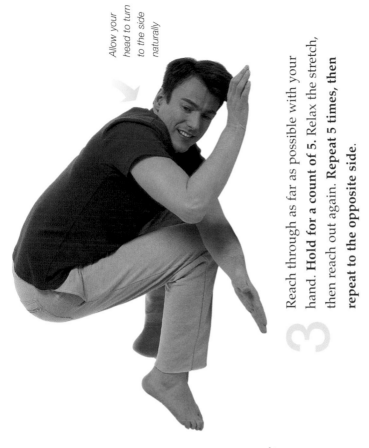

Allow your head to turn to the side naturally

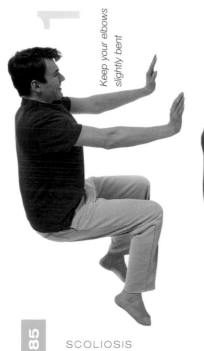

Keep your elbows slightly bent

Pull in your abs

1 Kneel on all fours with your hips directly above your knees, and your shoulders directly above your hands. Keep your back straight.

2 Lift one hand off the floor and slide it, palm up, along the floor between your other hand and knee. Bend the elbow of your supporting arm at the same time so that your free shoulder reaches toward the ground.

3 Reach through as far as possible with your hand. **Hold for a count of 5.** Relax the stretch, then reach out again. **Repeat 5 times, then repeat to the opposite side.**

MINI-PROGRAM

The exercise above is the most suitable isolated one for you to perform. Once you are comfortable with it, you should add more exercises to create a mini-program. Start with:

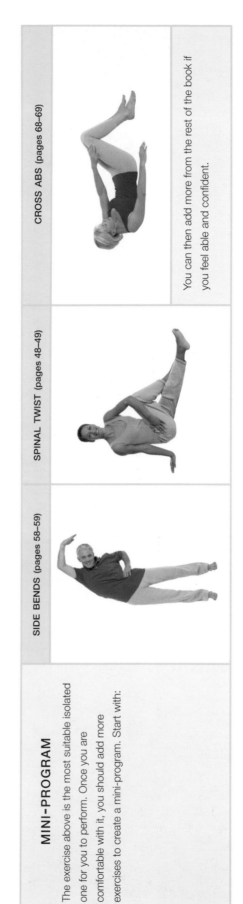

SIDE BENDS (pages 58–59)	SPINAL TWIST (pages 48–49)	CROSS ABS (pages 68–69)
		You can then add more from the rest of the book if you feel able and confident.

Osteoporosis

In osteoporosis the bones gradually lose their mineral content, become fragile, and can fracture easily. The main bones affected tend to be in the forearm, wrist, hip, and spine. Certain weight-bearing exercises can help prevent this.

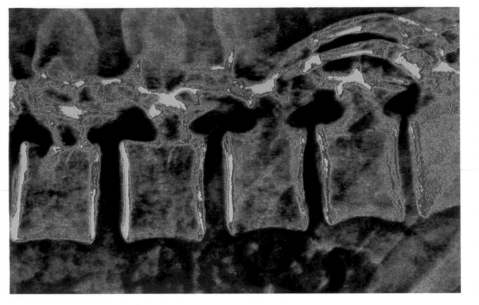

This is an X ray of vertebrae affected by osteoporosis. The dark patches within the orange vertebral bodies show the areas of decreased bone density. These, along with the biconcave invertebral spaces (blue), make the bone fragile.

Our skeleton is always making new cells and destroying old ones. These cells are made of minerals—primarily calcium—that make the bone hard. After the age of about 30, more cells tend to be lost than are created, so our bone mineral density (BMD) reduces, which can cause problems like osteoporosis. You may only realize you have osteoporosis if you incur a bone injury that seems out of proportion to your accident. Most at risk are people over 30 with a family history of the problem, or a personal history of eating disorders, and women who are menopausal, or have had a hysterectomy.

Osteoporosis causes the vertebrae to shrink, which can reduce a person's height by as much as 15 cm (6 in). If this occurs particularly in the thoracic spine, it can result in an exaggerated curve known as a "dowager's hump."

PREVENTION AND TREATMENT

- Seek your doctor's advice.
- Perform frequent short bursts of gentle, weight-bearing exercises, such as walking or light jogging.
- Eat a diet rich in calcium and vitamin D.

PURPOSE

The weight-bearing exercises below aim to increase bone mineral density and therefore bone strength and resilience by stimulating the bone to lay down more calcium and bone cells.

Is it right for me?

These activities are excellent for people of all back types. They are especially suitable for those who are at high risk of developing osteoporosis.

CAUTION

If you are at risk of osteoporosis, consult your doctor and have a bone mineral density scan before doing any high impact exercise. This will establish your susceptibility to fractures.

MINI-PROGRAM

The weight-bearing exercises on the left are the most effective. Once you are comfortable with them, you should begin to add more exercises to create a mini-program. Start with:

SIDE BENDS (pages 58–59)

PEC STRETCH (pages 60–61)

BACK EXTENDER (pages 66–67)

You can then add more from the rest of the book if you feel able and confident.

1 **Walking** is a good way to help prevent the onset of osteoporosis. If possible, walk up and down slopes. **Aim for at least a mile of walking at varied speeds, 3 times a week.** Make sure you maintain good posture throughout.

Keep your abs tight and your pelvis "tucked"

Try not to arch your back too much

2 **Jumping** up and down on the spot is good for your bones, too. **Jump for 5 minutes twice a day,** bending your knees as you land. Wear impact-reducing shoes when doing this.

Make sure you bend your knees on landing

3 **Jumping rope** is also effective. Start by skipping with the rope swinging backward, then change to forward. Finish in a backward direction to open up your shoulders and straighten your thoracic spine. **Gradually increase the length of time until you can skip for 10 minutes, twice a day, every other day.**

Professional Treatment

The majority of back problems respond to simple lifestyle changes such as good posture and regular exercise, but if the problem continues to interfere with your daily life, or worsens, you should consult your doctor.

MEDICAL ADVICE

Your doctor will take a full medical history, and examine your back for its range of movement, any tender spots, muscular weakness, or nerve involvement. Further investigations may be carried out to rule out or detect any more serious, underlying disorders.

You will then be advised on the medical treatment best for you. Options are as diverse as anti-inflammatory drugs and painkillers, tranquilizers to ease muscle spasm, a temporary corset to support the spine, or a referral to a particular type of treatment, such as physical therapy, osteopathy, or to a specialist. The latter three types of treatments are discussed in more detail below. Whichever course of action is recommended, it is important that you accompany it with an ongoing healthy lifestyle in order to keep your back the way you want it—in shape, and pain-free.

PHYSICAL THERAPY

Often a doctor's first choice, physical therapy deals with a wide range of problems. The treatments may include:

- localized manipulation and mobilization of the spine by the therapist;
- heat or cold treatments to ease muscle spasm and inflammation;
- traction—a longitudinal stretch performed manually or by rack-like equipment in order to relieve pressure on the spine;
- hydrotherapy;
- ultrasound treatments to reduce swelling, and promote the healing of soft tissues;
- tips for correct posture when standing, sitting, and doing everyday activities;

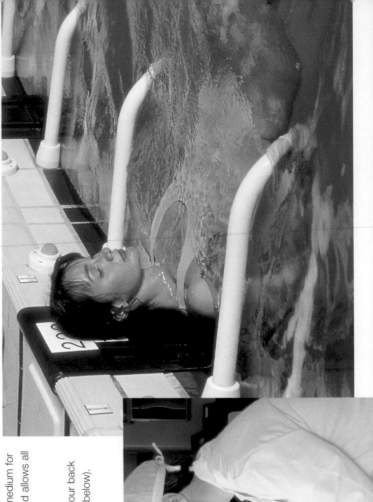

In hydrotherapy, water provides a medium for exercise that supports the body and allows all sorts of movement (right).

Your doctor may take an X ray of your back in case of certain spinal problems (below).

SPECIALISTS

If you are referred to a specialist such as an orthopedist, neurologist, or rheumatologist, you are likely to undergo further tests, such as a CAT scan (computerized axial tomography), which would show any central canal stenosis, a prolapsed disk, a fracture, or osteophyte formation (see pages 9–11 for explanations). Or you may have a discography to show whether there is any disk shrinkage, or prolapse: This is a type of X ray where you are injected with a radio opaque substance beforehand so that any problems will be easier to spot. Further medical recommendations will then be made based on the results of such tests. These may include:

■ an injection of corticosteroid into an inflamed joint by an anesthetist;

■ the removal, under anesthetic, of a prolapsed invertebral disk in order to relieve a trapped nerve root (discectomy); or

■ the removal, under anesthetic, of any osteophytes from around the facet joints or central canal (facetectomy).

OSTEOPATHY

This form of therapy was developed in 1874, and is an alternative to physical therapy. It is based on the belief that the misalignment of the spine is the main cause of back trouble, and therefore uses techniques to realign the spine. The techniques can help the common causes of chronic pain, but can be dangerous if the injury involves nerve damage.

■ recommendations on how to adapt your lifestyle at work and home;

■ advice on weight loss where necessary;

■ an exercise regime under the supervision of the therapist, with a daily home exercise program like the ones in this book.

An osteopath uses manual techniques, including pressure, stretching, and manipulation, to diagnose a problem, and restore healthy movements to the joints.

THE ALEXANDER TECHNIQUE

Developed in the mid-19th century by the actor F.M. Alexander, this technique for improving posture was based on his discovery that good posture helped reduce neck tension, thus greatly improving his performance on stage. Its aim is to eradicate what are known as "poor use" movements and posture, and to promote and maintain "good use" movements and posture. The paying student can be taught as part of a group, or individually. The Alexander technique is best for back pain caused by postural problems. It involves:

■ oral commands and hand pressure to re-educate poor posture and movement;

■ movements being broken down into their component parts;

■ repetition and practice until the correct movement "feels" right to the student.

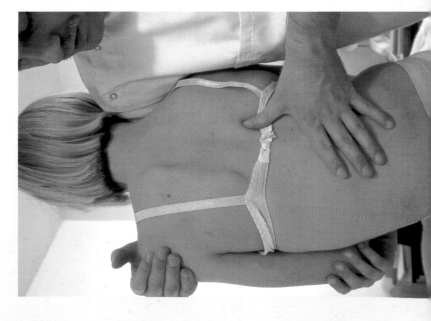

Home Treatments

There are many ways that you can help yourself when suffering from back pain. Simple home treatments can be integrated into your everyday routine, in addition to exercise programs like the ones in this book, or any medical advice or treatment you may be receiving.

You should remember that the pain you feel in your back is often out of proportion to the actual tissue damage incurred. This is because the muscles that support the spine tend to react to even the slightest excess strain by going into spasm. This affects the neighboring muscles, giving rise to tension and pain over a wide area, even though the actual point of damage may be only one facet joint, or disk. Some home treatments can effectively ease this muscle spasm, thus reducing the pain. These include:

MASSAGE

A massage can be of great help to ease away tension and pain. Make sure you choose a fully qualified masseur if you opt for a professional massage. Alternatively, you could use one of the many massage implements available to treat your own back. Or you could simply ask a friend to give you a gentle massage. The advice on the right should be followed to give a safe and effective massage.

You may find that a soothing massage from a kind friend is enough to alleviate your back pain. Find a comfortable position, and try dimming the lights and playing soft music so that you relax as much as possible.

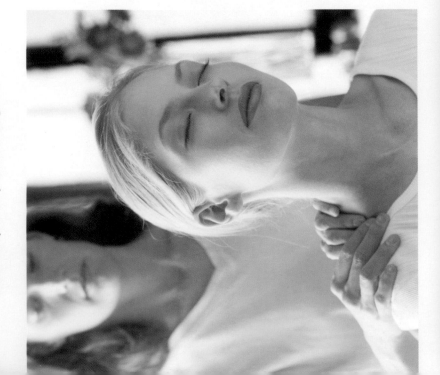

TIPS FOR GIVING MASSAGE

- Use a mild massage oil to prevent any friction when you begin the massage.
- Only massage the muscles on either side of the spine, not the spine itself; massaging the spine could do damage.
- Use the pad of your thumb to rub in small, circular motions.
- Always massage gently, and with control.
- Communicate with the person you are massaging so that you are aware of the pressure that he or she finds most comfortable.
- Concentrate on any "knots" you find in the muscles, until you feel them starting to loosen, or until your "patient's" discomfort starts to subside.

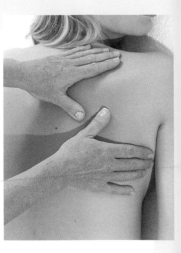

Another effective heat treatment to relieve muscle ache is simply to relax in a hot bath—complete with aromatic bubble bath, candles, and soft music for maximum relaxation.

PAINKILLERS

Over-the-counter painkillers often reduce pain. However, those that act as muscle relaxants as well, such as ibuprophen, are more beneficial. Never exceed the stated dose, and always ask advice if you are on other medication, or are pregnant. Never take painkillers long-term because you can end up requiring higher and higher doses to keep chronic pain under control (see box on the right for further information).

endorphins ("feel good" hormones), and block the slower-moving pain messages from reaching the brain, decreasing your discomfort.

REST

Bed rest is also a crucial part of the treatment for back pain as your back is under the least pressure when you are lying down. However, recent research has shown that prolonged bed rest can increase the chances of back problems recurring. It is now advised to take adequate rest, but to start exercising moderately as soon as possible after any back injury in order to speed long-term recovery.

HOW USEFUL ARE PAINKILLERS?

Endorphins are hormones released at certain times in your body that override the sensation of pain. As painkillers are made to mimic the effect of endorphins, your body thinks it has a sufficient supply of them when painkillers are taken on a regular basis, and ceases to produce its own. This makes your body incapable of dulling pain on its own, which means that your chronic pain may return even worse than before if you stop taking the painkillers. It is therefore all-too-easy to become reliant on them. It is not recommended to take painkillers on a long-term basis, although occasional use to relieve extreme pain is certainly acceptable.

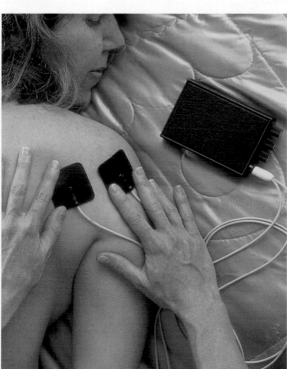

A TENS machine is easy to use to relieve discomfort: place the electrodes on your skin, and use the dials to adjust the frequency and strength of the electrical impulses you receive.

HOT AND COLD TREATMENTS

When your back feels particularly painful, use heat- and cold-sprays, or muscle lotions on the problem area. Alternatively, press a hot water bottle, or a covered ice pack against your back. Cold treatments are best to treat swelling, while hot treatments are better for easing muscle spasm. These treatments do not affect the muscles themselves, but instead block out the hot or cold sensation before the feeling of pain.

SUPPORTS

A neck or back brace, available at specialist stores, should only ever be used as a temporary measure because long-term use would allow the muscles to weaken from underuse, worsening the problem in the long-run.

TENS MACHINE

TENS stands for Transcutaneous Electrical Nerve Stimulation. You use a TENS machine by placing the pads attached to it onto your back. It transmits little pulses of electrical energy into your body, which stimulate the production of

Lifestyle Hints

Your daily activities have a great impact on your back. For example, DIY, housework, and gardening can be good for your back, but can place unnecessary stress on it if carried out incorrectly. Only do a little at a time, and always take regular breaks.

RECOMMENDED ACTIVITIES

Yoga and other eastern exercise routines, such as tai chi, are an excellent way of improving flexibility, and reducing stresses. As with any exercise routine, never attempt too much too quickly. If you have an existing back problem,

or have had trouble with your back, always tell your instructor before joining a class as there are certain advanced exercises that are not suitable for people with back problems.

Swimming is also a popular method of exercising and strengthening your back. The water reduces the effects of gravity, so that the muscles can work without tension, and the joints can bend and stretch without pressure. Swimming tones the back and stomach muscles, eases muscle spasms, and increases flexibility. Backstroke is particularly effective as it helps open up the chest and shoulders, and therefore counteracts poor posture.

Walking is another effective yet low-risk form of exercise that can help bad backs. Maintain good posture while walking, and always wear comfortable, fully supporting shoes.

All types of sports are an excellent way to keep fit and reduce stress, but only if they are played regularly, and sensibly. Avoid sudden bursts of strenuous activity. It is important to have the appropriate clothing and equipment for whatever sports you undertake.

Yoga classes are a popular way of remaining fit, strong, and healthy, as well as relieving stress. You can also practice yoga moves at home on your own.

When out walking, carry items like your water bottle and waterproof coat in a backpack so that all weight is evenly distributed.

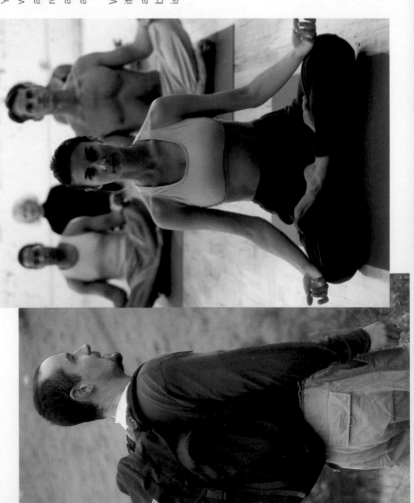

✓ GOOD PRACTICE

EXERCISE REGULARLY at a level appropriate to your fitness ability.

DO YOUR BACK EXERCISE ROUTINE REGULARLY in order to maintain strong stomach and back muscles, and a flexible spine.

MAINTAIN THE CORRECT WEIGHT FOR YOUR HEIGHT (see advice on Body Mass Index, right) as being overweight increases stress on the spine, especially if the weight is carried around your midriff.

CHECK YOUR POSTURE at frequent intervals—whether sitting or standing. The crown of your head should be the tallest part of your body, your neck and back should be in a neutral position, and you should aim to have a slight pelvic tilt (see page 8).

MAKE SURE YOU GET A GOOD NIGHT'S SLEEP EVERY NIGHT, and take naps, if necessary, to refresh yourself. Lying down flat is the only position that rests the back.

USE CORRECT LIFTING TECHNIQUES (see page 20). Bend your knees, not your back, to pick up heavy objects. Make sure that the loads are distributed evenly between the two sides of the body, and are carried close to you.

WEAR SENSIBLE, COMFORTABLE SHOES, especially when doing any weight-bearing exercise.

✗ BAD PRACTICE

DON'T OVEREAT as this may lead to excess weight, which increases the pressure on your spine.

STEER CLEAR OF SNOOZING IN ARMCHAIRS as sitting increases the pressure on your lower spine and therefore does not allow your back to relax.

AVOID WEARING HIGH HEELS as they cause the curve at the base of the spine to be accentuated. This not only compresses the lumbar vertebrae but also throws the body's center of gravity off balance.

AVOID ANY STATIC POSITION that puts your back muscles under strain for a long time, like bending over the tub to wash your hair, or ironing. Instead, find a comfortable position to do these in or try to prop one foot on a bar or foot rest while doing them.

TRY NOT TO CARRY BAGS ON ONE SIDE ONLY—instead carry one in each hand, or if carrying only one, alternate sides throughout the day, especially with shoulder bags.

TRY NOT TO LET YOURSELF SLOUCH when standing, walking, or sitting.

AVOID DOING TWO MOVEMENTS AT ONCE, such as bending down and twisting to the side.

BODY MASS INDEX (BMI)

Find out whether you are of a suitable weight for your height by calculating your body mass index (BMI):

Multiply your weight in pounds by 705, divide this by your height in inches, then divide again by your height in inches.
eg: Weight (W) = 146 pounds
Height (H) = 67 inches
$146(W) \times 705 = 102\,930$
$102\,930 \div 67(H) \div 67(H) = 23$
$BMI = 23$
Then consult the chart below.

BMI	ADVICE
19–25	Your weight is not excessive for your height, and is unlikely to be placing too great a stress on your back and joints.
25–30	Your BMI suggests that you are overweight. In addition to possible heart and circulation problems, you are likely to be placing a significant strain on your back. Exercise your back muscles, and maintain good posture to lessen the risk of injury.
Above 30	A BMI of 30 or above is considered obese. If you do not already suffer from back problems, it is likely that you soon will. Back exercise will help prevent injury, but losing weight is essential.

Glossary

ABDUCTORS Muscles that move a joint away from the body.

ADDUCTORS Muscles that move a joint toward the body.

CARTILAGE A hard but flexible substance that forms part of the skeleton, together with bone. It lines the ends of bones at the joints and, together with fibrous tissue, forms the intervertebral disks of the spine.

CAT SCAN A Computerized Axial Tomography Scan involves cross-sectional images of the body produced by computer analysis of a series of X rays.

COSTO-VERTEBRAL JOINT The joint between a rib and a vertebra.

EXTENSORS Muscles that straighten, or extend, a joint.

FACET JOINT One of four joints on each vertebra that connects the vertebra with its upper and lower neighbors.

FLEXORS Muscles that bend a joint.

HIGH IMPACT EXERCISE Exercise in which a joint absorbs the stress of landing on the ground during movement, such as jogging, skipping, and jumping.

INVERTEBRAL DISK A pad, made of cartilage and fibrous tissue with a fluid center, that lies between each vertebral body and acts as a shock absorber.

INVERTEBRAL SPACE The opening on each side of a vertebra.

JOINT The site at which bones meet and move against each other.

LIGAMENT A strong band of fibrous tissue that binds bones together at joints.

MUSCLE A tissue that can contract and relax, either to cause movement or support the body structure.

NEURAL OR SPINAL ARCH A bony column, made of all the vertebrae, that contains and protects the spinal cord.

NEURAL CANAL The tube-like space surrounded by the neural arch.

NEUROLOGIST A medical or surgical specialist concerned with disorders affecting the nervous system.

MUSCLES AND BONES: BACK VIEW

This diagram shows the position of the main bones and muscles of the back mentioned in the book. Common names are given in parentheses.

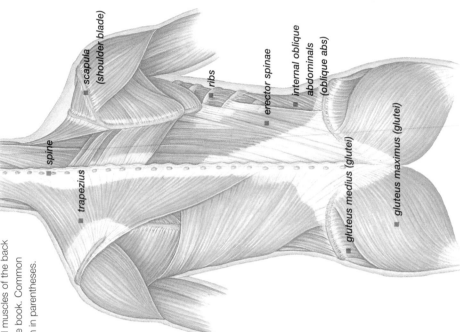

- trapezius
- spine
- scapula (shoulder blade)
- ribs
- erector spinae
- internal oblique abdominals (oblique abs)
- gluteus medius (glutei)
- gluteus maximus (glutei)

MUSCLES AND BONES: FRONT VIEW

This diagram shows the position of the major bones and muscles on the front side of the body that are mentioned in the book. Common names are given in parentheses.

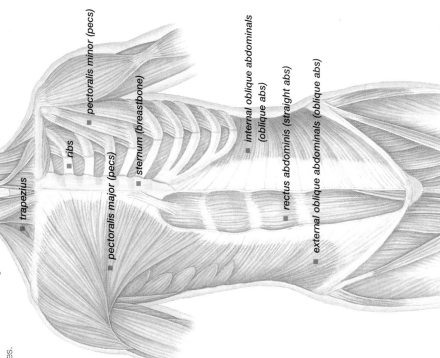

- trapezius
- ribs
- pectoralis minor (pecs)
- sternum (breastbone)
- pectoralis major (pecs)
- internal oblique abdominals (oblique abs)
- rectus abdominis (straight abs)
- external oblique abdominals (oblique abs)

"NEUTRAL" POSITION OF THE BACK, NECK, HEAD, OR CHIN A posture in which all the curves of the spinal column are held in their natural and correct position.

ORTHOPEDIST A specialist in the treatment of skeletal disorders.

OSTEOPATHY A therapy consisting of physical manipulation of the bones, based on the belief that this will restore proper function to the skeleton and other tissues.

OSTEOPHYTES Bony spurs that develop inside or at the edges of a joint due to wear and tear, often causing osteoarthritis.

PELVIC "TUCK" The position when the base of the pelvis is tilted forward and the lower back is flattened. This pose should be adopted at the start of each exercise.

PHYSICAL THERAPY A form of therapy that uses measures as varied as exercise, manipulation, heat, and hydrotherapy to treat people with all kinds of disorders.

POSTURAL MUSCLES Muscles that help you maintain posture.

RHEUMATOLOGIST A specialist in conditions involving inflammation and pain in the muscles, joints, and fibrous tissue.

ROTATORS Muscles that turn a joint in a circular movement.

SPINAL CORD The lower section of the central nervous system, which runs from the base of the brain down through the neural canal to the lumbar vertebrae, and tapers off into a fine thread. Throughout the cord's course, nerve roots branch off through the intervertebral spaces.

SPINOUS PROCESS A large bony spur that projects from the back of the neural arch and provides attachments for ligaments and muscles.

TRANSVERSE PROCESS A bony spur that sticks out on each side of the spinal arch and provides a point of attachment for the spinal ligaments and muscles.

VERTEBRA(E) The 33 small bones that form the spine.

VERTEBRAL BODY The thick, rounded area of bone on the front of each vertebra.

WEIGHT-BEARING EXERCISE Exercise in which a joint takes the weight of the body during movement, such as walking and jogging.

Index

ACKNOWLEDGMENTS

I would like to thank Nigel Perryman for his "constructive" criticism, which made this a better book, despite somewhat ruining the schedule; his son, Tom Perryman, who was coerced into doing many of the exercises before I would produce his supper; and Wuss Jones, who put up with me prodding his back when he should have been working on my bathroom! More seriously, I am most grateful to Kelly Thompson, my editor, for her unfailing humor, professionalism, and attention to detail, and to Jules Selmes, an excellent photographer who allowed me many sneaky breaks during photo shoots, and flattered me out of my attempts to become one of the models.

Picture Credits

6 (right) SPL, 7 (far left) BSIP DR. T. Pichard/SPL, 9 GJLP/SPL, 82 Scott Camazine, Sue Trainor/SPL, 86 Alfred Pasieka/SPL, 88 (center) Ouellette & Theroux, Publicphoto Diffusion/SPL, 88 (right) BSIP CH Themale Soiel/SPL, 89 Hattie Young//SPL, 91 Dan McCoy/Rainbow/Medipics

SPL = Science Photo Library
Picture Researcher Sandra Schneider